True POWER Of HYDROGEN PEROXIDE

Miracle Path to Wellness

By Mary Wright

Warning Disclaimers:

The information in this book is presented as a matter of general interest only and not as prescribing cures. Readers must use their own judgment; consult their qualified medical expert, or their personal licensed physician for specific applications to their individual health issues. The author and publisher assume no responsibility for error, inaccuracies, or any inconsistency herein.

This book is for general information purposes only and is not intended as a substitute for medical advice. You should consult with a physician or other healthcare professional familiar with nutrition, prevention, and related health issues. No statement in this book has been approved by or been evaluated or certified by the Food and Drug Administration (FDA). Statements in this book are not intended to diagnose, treat, cure or prevent any disease. Always consult your qualified medical practitioner prior to using any substance or product for any medical condition including any product mentioned or offered here. The FDA has not approved of the usage of hydrogen peroxide for any medical purpose.

Library of Congress Cataloging-In-Publication Date
Power of Hydrogen Peroxide
Bibliography and Index
ISBN: 978-0-615-95149-2
PowerOfHydrogenPeroxide@gmail.com

PowerOfHydrogenPeroxide.com

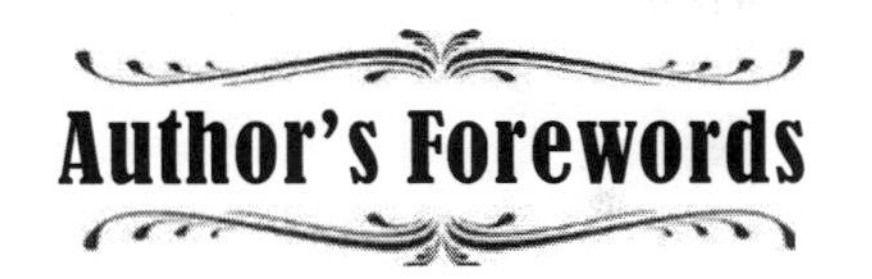

Author's Forewords

These are exciting times with all the discoveries of new alternative health options and paths to wellness. It was many years ago that I first questioned what is true healthcare, what causes and cures illness and disease, and what options and alternatives are available. The list is long and I personally explored and researched many.

My initial skepticism was quickly dispersed. Most exciting was discovering and developing an understanding of the incredible potentials of hydrogen peroxide, one of the simplest natural substances and most incredible substances containing 2 of the 4 essentials of life: water and oxygen.

More wondrous is that that is all that hydrogen peroxide is. Pure water. Pure oxygen. The core of hydrogen peroxide's working element is pure oxygen. Oxygen equals life.

This book is next in the evolution of books on the topic bringing the subject up to date by both explanations in understandable terms and realistic, affordable and practical potential applications. This book is not a recital of prior books or a reprint ing of any outdated book.

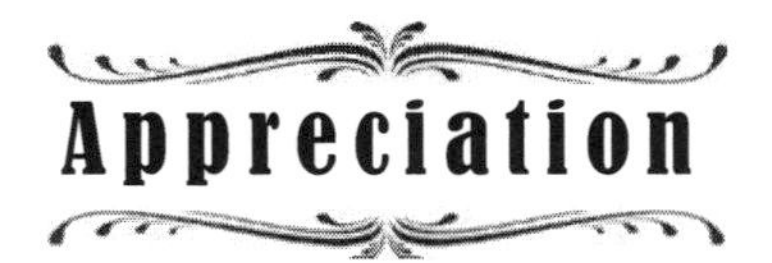

Appreciation

Over the years so many people have contributed to the evolution and advancement of knowledge and information about hydrogen peroxide and therapy. Many people including those that I personally know have benefited by their efforts and information sharing.

I could not begin to express my true sincere appreciation to the many individuals, healthcare professionals, medical experts and researchers in health and wellness fields who contributed to and assisted in this book to bring forth understanding and practical applications of oxygenation, hydrogen peroxide therapy, the many usages of hydrogen peroxide, and the overall field of cellular nutrient supplementing.

This book represents decades of efforts by countless people across the world leading to today. This book is possible by their ongoing efforts and by those who directly and in information sharing contribute their wisdom, experience, research and expertise for this book. No words could fully express my personal appreciation for your contributions.

Thank you.

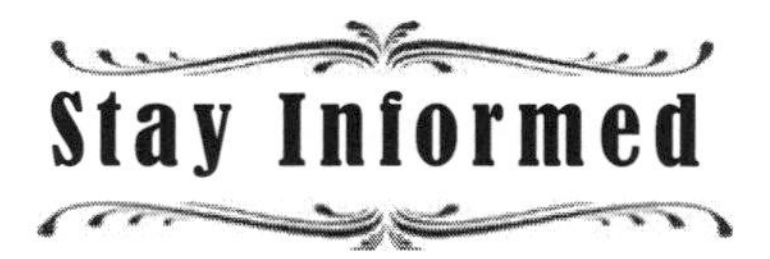

Stay Informed

Most books on alternative personal healthcare and wellness topics are merely rehashing and rewriting earlier books. The information may be decades old, outdated and incomplete. An identical replacement book is then reprinted year after year with nothing new in the content.

Unlike most other books on personal wellness through personal healthh decisions and action, which tend to grind on redundantly – only to urge mega- dosing on a single dietary supplement, pill or liquid as the magic solution - this book considers and presents in real, useable and affordable ways how to obtain whole body cellular health and true wellness.

For example, one currently popular book on hydrogen peroxide often sold was actually first published in 1991 – over two decades ago. For the most part, it complains about government agencies, corporate healthcare and drug companies. It repeats itself redundantly page after page on the topic and finally gets to the point, which is to only urges mega-dosing with one supplement. That book has been republished over and over and over. The author passed away years ago, but the book company kept reprinting.

While it contained worthwhile information, the amount of new professional and legitimate research by laboratories, biochemists, and licensed medical researchers willing to step outside the box has been extensive and with new discovery after discovery worldwide.

True Power of Hydrogen Peroxide, Miracle Path to Wellness 2014 is not a reprinting of an old book. This is a new publication, not a repeat of any older book. The only way to produce a truly up-to-date book is to start fresh and from the beginning.

The exploration and research on how the human body works, what prevents and cures diseases and how to maximize physical health and mental focus is being undertaken worldwide by the most brilliant minds and qualified researchers who are willing to not be limited by conventional establishment wisdom. Information sharing by all of us is vital to maximizing learning and benefiting from our experiences, knowledge and investigation.

This Book Is A Living Book.

This book will be updated, edited and printed quarterly to allow continual updating, corrections and clarifications.

Updates will be available to you on any materials in new updates to this book free of charge if you wish. In this way it is a living book that is evolving in knowledge-sharing as more information is learned and better understood. This will be shared with you making this a living book to you.

As the author I invite you to contact me by email if you wish to receive updates on new information and practical application of topics of this book and new knowledge of whole health wellness.

Share your Experiences & Knowledge With Others.

If you learn of additional information or have your own experiences you believe others could learn from and wish to be shared, I would encourage you to drop me an email with your information. If your material is used in subsequent printings, let me know in your email whether you wish acknowledgement in the book or bibliography, or wish to remain anonymous. A PhD is not required for you to be knowledgeable, know information by your personal health experiences or to have valuable information to share with others.

Help Write This Book.

Each printing of this book will be updated with new information, additional clarifications and needed corrections. You can help spread and improve the knowledge and quality of how it is presented.

Abuse This Book.

Abuse this book, not your body. Fold the corners, write and doodle all over it, highlight what is useful to you, and make your notes on the blank backs of pages and inside the cover.

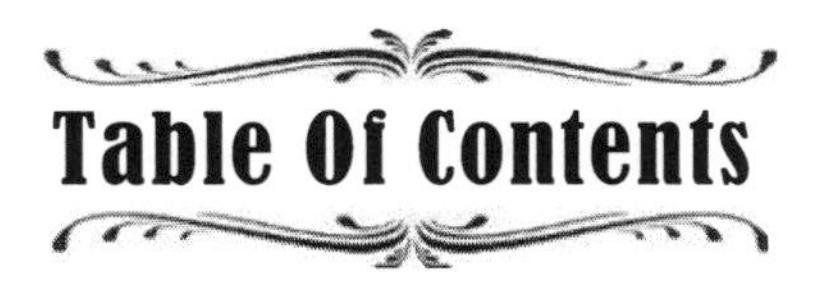

Table Of Contents

Appreciation iii

Author's Foreword v

Stay Informed vii

Chapter 1 What is Oxygen? 1

Chapter 2 What is Hydrogen Peroxide? 3

Chapter 3 What Does Food Grade Mean? 5

Chapter 4 Why 35%? 7

Chapter 5 Benefits of Super-Oxygenation 9

Chapter 6 The Dangers of Cells Lacking Sufficient Oxygen........ 11

Chapter 7 Hydrogen Peroxide Protects & Restores Wellness ... 17

- How does the body receive oxygen?
- Oxygen and essential nutrients through our skin
- Oxygen & essential nutrients through food & stomach
- Lungs intake and expel oxygen and toxins

Chapter 8 Obesity on the Rise 23

Chapter 9 Hydrogen Peroxide Oxygen Therapy 27

- Through your skin
- Through your mouth
- Through your Digestive System

Chapter 10 Oral Super-Oxygenation 31

- Week 1 Thru Week 3
- Allowing Your Body to Set Your Protocol
- What is Chelation Therapy

Chapter 11 Reducing Hydrogen Peroxide Concentration 37

Chapter 12 Essential Cellular and Body Support 39

Chapter 13 Removing Toxins From Home: Chlorine 41

- Known Chlorine Dangers
- Known Bromine Dangers
- Dangers of combining Chlorine and Bromine
- Protect your children and grandchildren
- How dangerous is?
- Vapor dangers
- Priorities & Economics of Personal Health
- The Body's Natural-Defensive Smell Factor

Chapter 14 Hydrogen Peroxide for Pool, Hot Tub & Bath 51

- Spa Usage and Costs
- Pond Maintenance
- Safety Comparison
- Pool Side Plant Health

Chapter 15 Removing Chemicals From Home: Aromatics 59

Chapter 16 Decline in Food Quality 63

- Minerals your cells need
- How obtain essential trace minerals

Chapter 17 Hydrogen Peroxide In Bathwater 65

- Hydrogen Peroxide works against Micro-organisms
- What to add to bath water

Chapter 18 The Benefits of Magnesium 69

Chapter 19 Single Supplement Mega-dosing? 87

- Maximized Cellular Oxygen & Nutrient Balance
- Allow Your Cellular Body A Day Of Rest

Chapter 20 Natural Sea Salts ....,,,............ 91

- Best Sea Salt
- Himalayan Salt
- Dead Sea Salt
- How to consider health & Wellness

Chapter 21 Storage of Hydrogen Peroxide 99

- Personal Safety
- Store Safely
- Store in Dark
- Store in Refrigerator or Cool Location
- How Long Hydrogen Peroxide Lasts

Chapter 22 Many Uses Of Hydrogen Peroxide 103

- Internal Usage (also see Chapter 9)
- Swimming Pool & Hot Tub
- Fruits & Vegetables
- Hand Wash
- Meats
- Houseplants
- Home Sanitizing
- For Laundry
- Dish Water
- Use in Bath Tub
- Pets & Pet's Water
- Aquarium
- Foot Bath and Sterilizing
- Mouthwash
- Internal Usage Warning

Chapter 23 Personal Wellness Checklist 111

- Read this Chapter for full list

Chapter 24 Listen To Your Cellular Body.............................. 115

Chapter 25 Food For Thought 121

Chapter 26 The Importance Of Balance 129

Author's Closing Comment 131

Bibliography 133

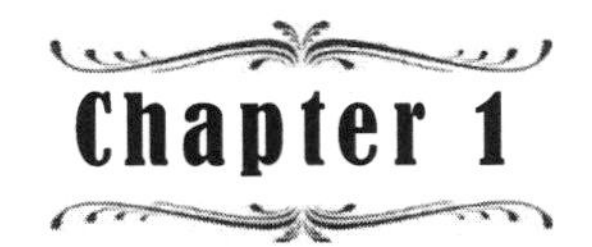

Chapter 1

What is Oxygen?

Oxygen is a gaseous element. It is shown in chemical charts with the symbol O. It the most abundant element on earth and is colorless, odorless and tasteless.

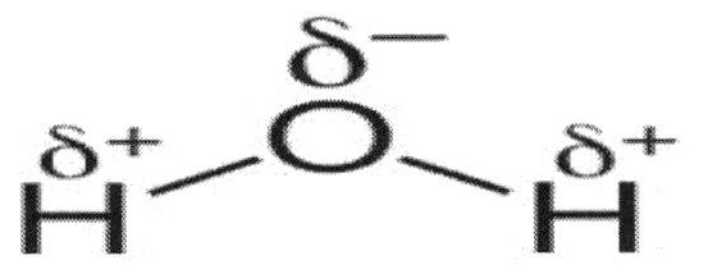

90% of water, over half of the human body and only approximately 20% of the air we breathe is oxygen.

The typical reaction of oxygen when joined with other substances is oxidation. Oxidation is a chemical reaction with many various results. In the human body, it converts or burns sugar into energy. Oxygen helps to remove wastes from the human body. Oxidation can purify and sterilize. Oxidation is an exceptionally powerful defense against pathogens.

The natural element of oxygen (02) is 1 of the 4 elements of life: oxygen, hydrogen, nitrogen and carbon.

Incredibly, hydrogen peroxide contains two of those elements. These 4 elements are the essentials of life and the most urgent. Without oxygen, our bodies and our cells quickly die. In a medical emergency, the most common immediately medical response is to administer oxygen.

Having a sufficient supply of oxygen to our cells is absolutely critical. Oxygen starvation may be the greatest cause of degenerative diseases. The declining level of oxygen in the air we breathe, which also increasingly contains pathogens, harmful micro-organism and toxins, is what most contributes to the seeming rapid increase in degenerative diseases. This is worsened by the lack of nutritious and healthy diets – all constituting continual depravation, starvation and assault against our body and the cells of our body.

Oxygen powers our body the way a motor requires oxygen to run. A

1

supercharged motor produces more power because more oxygen is forced through it. To reduce oxygen to the human body is to reduce its power, including curative power, energy levels and cell reproduction. To enhance oxygen has the opposite beneficial effects.

In the right concentration, oxygen maximizes the healing process, the immune system and disease prevention. Every cellular, organ and body function requires oxygen, which is carried throughout the human body by blood as the method of acquiring this necessity.

Oxygen also is vital to beneficial aerobic bacteria within the human body. However oxygen also is destructive of harmful anaerobic bacteria that are found in the environment, contaminated food and impure water – and that invade our bodies. Oxygen is the natural method to prevent and destroy anaerobic bacteria within our bodies.

Oxygen is the most essential element of life and wellness.

Chapter 2

What is Hydrogen Peroxide?

Water is h2o. That means in has two atoms of hydrogen and one atom of oxygen. Hydrogen peroxide has an extra oxygen atom. Hydrogen peroxide has the symbol h2o2.

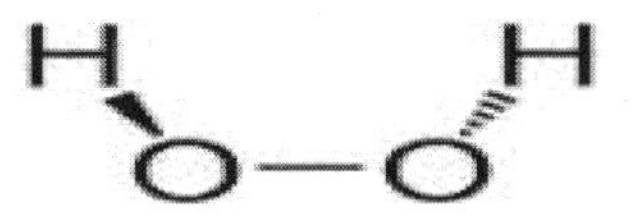

That additional "O" – the extra oxygen atom - is the working element of hydrogen peroxide - a pure oxygen atom. It is that extra oxygen atom that is the miracle of hydrogen peroxide because that pure oxygen atom can be released. It is the oxygen atom that is the benefit. Its' power cannot be understated in both preserving and protecting human life.

First, we need to understand what hydrogen peroxide is. It is a very simple, pure substance. Water is designated as h2o, while hydrogen peroxide chemically is designated as h2o2. Specifically, this means hydrogen peroxide is water with an extra pure oxygen atom.

Hydrogen peroxide is colorless, slightly heavier than water, and has a distinct taste. Hydrogen peroxide is only a semi-stable substance, which is necessary to how hydrogen peroxide works.

Heat will cause hydrogen peroxide to release one of its two oxygen atoms. When hydrogen peroxide comes in contact with certain organic substances, certain minerals, certain chemicals and with the enzyme catalase it breaks down the hydrogen peroxide.

When hydrogen peroxide breaks down (called decomposition) releasing one of the two oxygen atoms. It becomes pure water and pure oxygen – h2o and 0. This pure oxygen is very powerful as the decomposition also releases energy. This also is the reason hydrogen peroxide is so beneficial.

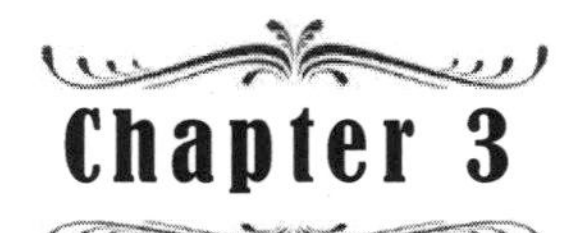

Chapter 3

What Does "Food Grade" Mean?

There are dozens of grades and types of hydrogen peroxide offered commercially. Hydrogen peroxide is one of the most commonly used of all chemicals. Over 99% of hydrogen peroxide is used for industrial manufacturing and processing.

The purity and health safety of hydrogen peroxide for manufacturing and processing does not matter for such industrial uses. Because of this, the priority in making industrial hydrogen peroxide is to minimize production costs and to maximize its stability, storage life and for resistance against heat and cold. As a result, little concern is given to its purity and many forms of stabilizers, heavy metals and other additives are used to obtain those goals. Many of those additives and stabilizers are extremely destructive to the human body.

Hydrogen peroxide also is used in the food industry for processing, sterilizing, and cleaning. For this reason, industry, laboratories and government agencies have set a standard and inspection/testing protocol for hydrogen peroxide before it can be certified, used and marketed as being specifically "food grade."

Specifically, "food grade" means that the hydrogen peroxide is certified to meet government and industry standards for being used with food. As a result, it is an assurance that it does not have contaminants, toxins, cancer-causing and toxic heavy metals and other harmful ingredients.

Why would anyone sell non-food grade falsely claiming it is? There are many reasons. The foremost reason is that it costs far less to buy industrial hydrogen peroxide. Cheap industrial hydrogen peroxide also is more stable, so is easier to store for a long period of time and is more stable for shipping. They will even often boast their hydrogen peroxide can be stored in a super cold freezer and it won't freeze. This is because it is not food grade and therefore has chemicals in it that serve to act like anti-freeze. Pure hydrogen peroxide has a higher freezing point than 100% water, but it will freeze.

The percentage of concentration indicates the percentage that is hydrogen peroxide. So 8% means the ingredients are 8% hydrogen peroxide and 92% water. 35% means the ingredients are 35% hydrogen peroxide. The balance is water.

For that reason, putting true certified 35% food grade hydrogen peroxide in the freezer can alter the concentration level and cause separation because food grade hydrogen peroxide has no harmful chemicals to act as stabilizers and anti-freeze.

From a consumer's view, this makes what seems good hydrogen peroxide for health and wellness usage counter intuitive. But in fact if the hydrogen will not freeze at very cold temperature, if the bottle never swells building up pressure, and overall seems very stable, this indicates that it is not food grade and must not be consumed, used with food or used in any other way that may interact with your body.

35% food grade hydrogen peroxide offers many oxygenation and anti-microbial benefits. 35% food grade hydrogen peroxide is the only form of hydrogen peroxide to use for health and home.

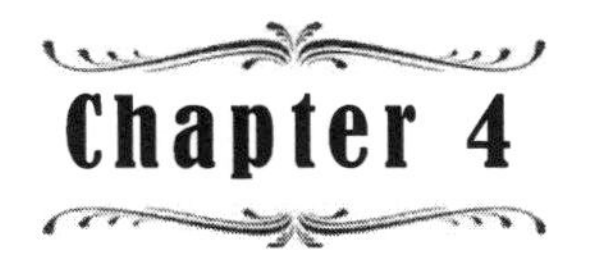

Chapter 4

Why 35 %?

35% means that the liquid is 35% hydrogen peroxide and 65% water. There is no such thing as a bottle of 100% hydrogen peroxide. It is impossible to manufacture. Even the military can only make 90% concentration hydrogen peroxide and that will decompose very quickly.

35% is the highest concentration that can be sold to consumers and the highest concentration that can be shipped to consumers.

All classic, professional and legitimate research materials and health publications have always specifically referred only to 35% food grade hydrogen peroxide and no other concentration level. There is a specific reason.

The only true food grade hydrogen peroxide manufactured in the United States is in 35% and 50% concentration. It is only produced in a very limited number of monitored and certified refiners, with the quality and purity checked by government inspectors to be devoid of certain harmful additives, heavy metals and stabilizers that are extremely destructive to the human body.

There is no such thing as homemade or small scale production of hydrogen peroxide.

Unfortunately, for many reasons mostly related to cost, numerous individuals, websites, and merchants now offer hydrogen peroxide they claim is food grade when it is not. Food grade hydrogen peroxide, whether in bulk, wholesale or retail, costs much more to produce and buy. They claim there is no difference when in fact the difference could slowly destroy your health or just be falsely labeled the bottles. Because they sell other than 35% food grade, they declare it is irrelevant.

They know that you cannot taste the different and the price seemingly is lower. But destroying your health is not worth the savings and it unlikely you are saving money. It takes 450% as much 8% hydrogen peroxide to equal 35%, plus what you would pay in shipping for each 8% order.

Worse, regardless of what they have on the label, it is not food grade. Generally, if you research you also will find such individuals and companies have been in business and online for a very short period of time.

Hydrogen peroxide is used in numerous areas of manufacturing, sterilizing, cleaning, bleaching, and in the food industry. If it is for manufacturing, the primary concerns are keeping the costs low and with long term storage ability. For retail sales in stores, non-food grade is preferred as it remains stable longer on the shelf. Not strictly purifying the hydrogen peroxide plus using other chemicals and stabilizers in manufacturing and storage of the hydrogen peroxide dramatically reduces the costs. However, this also is the reason only 35% food grade hydrogen peroxide should be used for health therapy, used internally, used for any contact with your skin, food or in your home, pool or other human contact ways.

If you review any of the true scientific and medical research materials dating back decades you find that all specifically and only discuss and recommend 35% food grade hydrogen peroxide.

Chapter 5

Benefits of Super-Oxygenation

A Healthy Outside Comes From The Inside

Oxygen is the most critical cellular body need. A person can live for days without water and weeks without food. But within minutes your body, cells and brain are permanently damaged without oxygen.

The level of oxygen in the air we breathe historically has been dropping. In some areas it is as low as 19%. In urban areas it is lower – dropping to as low as 10%. Added to the air we breathe are increasing levels of all the toxins and contaminants, dust, pathogens, fungus, bacteria and viruses. Many people have less than perfect lungs due to years or decades of pollutants, smoke damage, and other environmental and aging effects that reduce lung efficiency.

Simple common sense tells us that having a well oxygenated body is critical to good health, a good immune system, and sufficient energy levels. Super-oxygenation addresses the question of whether a person's cells are receiving sufficient oxygen. Sufficient oxygen is vital for optimum health in today's contaminated world as oxygen levels decline.

Oxygen is of utmost importance. Oxygen powers our cells, cleans our blood and body, destroys harmful micro-organisms, maximizes body strength, and is vital for optimum brain function.

How does the body take in oxygen? Three ways:

1. Through the lungs

2. Through the skin

3. Through the stomach

You may have heard about directly injecting oxygen into the body. This is called "intravenous" use of hydrogen peroxide. Is this safe to do yourself? No. Directly injecting h2o2 into your body can be destructive or lethal if not done perfectly by a qualified doctor or health professional.

Pure oxygen is a very powerful and in direct, excessive contact can be very damaging. Your body has to process the oxygen through one of the three methods above before entering the blood stream. If not it, can damage the body and develop air bubbles to potentially block the blood stream.

If oxygen is so important, why isn't it more advocated? In fact, most of you know that in a medical trauma the first thing an EMT team and medical staff often will do is administer oxygen. It is understood to be that important to life – especially in a medical crisis.

Oxygen therapy has been around for a long time. Hydrogen peroxide was discovered in the early 1800s. It was first used as an antiseptic because of the ability of oxygen (which is what hydrogen peroxide releases) to destroy viruses, harmful bacteria and fungus.

3% was a concentration level determined not to harm the skin. 3% hydrogen peroxide became the first working mouth wash to kill the bacteria in a person's mouth that causes bad breathe. It became the primary way to sterilize kitchens, food processing and surgical tools.

The simple element of oxygen is a powerful anti-bacterial, anti-fungus and anti-virus weapon. Oxygen therapy has been around for a long time. Hippocrates, called "The Father Of Medicine," vehemently urged his patients to breathe fresh open air, not the musty air of a closed room. Yet now we sleep in sealed houses with no fresh air flow, further reducing oxygen during vital recuperative sleep. His #1 medicine? Oxygen.

This also is understood in animal husbandry and livestock. Even in the coldest climates, barns and sheds generally have open windows to the South to allow fresh air. If not, the animals will quickly become sick, contract pneumonia, and become weak and infected.

Viruses do not live long in a ventilated room; but will blossom in a closed environment.

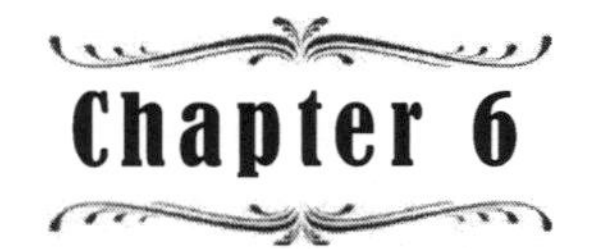

Chapter 6

Dangers of Cells Lacking Sufficient Oxygen?

People's bodies are receiving less oxygen than in the past and less than what nature intended for us. There are many reasons why we now have less oxygen:

- The oxygen level in the air has declined.
- Food we eat has less oxygen in it.
- Air pollution.

Lung damage from pollution, smoking, and breathing bad air.

Closed air conditioning and heating systems that recirculate increasingly lower oxygen content air.

Sealing homes and business for energy efficiency that prevents fresh air, which causes the oxygen content to increasingly decline in your home, while carbon monoxide and micro-organism count increases.

Lack of physical activity for which our heart and lungs are weaker and pumping less oxygen, plus contaminated air causes lungs to slow.

In a real sense, many people are continually suffocating at less than the level of oxygen their blood, cells and brain needs. The effect in the long-run is cumulative and ultimately is health-devastating.

Oxygen not only powers the cells of our body, it has essential and powerful curative and preventative abilities. In addition to destroying viruses, harmful bacteria, and fungus, it also assists to remove carbon monoxide from the body.

When a person has COPD *(lung disease)* the problem is not just a lack of the lungs taking in enough oxygen. But there also is a problem that the body cannot expel enough carbon monoxide, which is a deadly poison. This also causes rapid cell deterioration and weakens the immune system, allowing pathogens to invade and cause illness and disease.

Lack of sufficient oxygen for your blood and cells is accumulatively destructive. This continually weakens the human body, cells, and the immune system. Energy levels and mental alertness drop. The body increasingly builds up wastes and toxins it cannot remove. The scale can then finally be tripped allowing the person to contract a major illness, tumor, degenerative disease, mental illness, suffer a heart attack or stroke and become infected with a deadly virus or bacterial disease.

The lack of sufficient oxygen will allow or cause our cellar wellness to be attacked, damaged and weakened. This might be the liver or kidneys, lungs or heart, lymphoid glands, brain or nervous system, stomach or eyes, hearing or sense of smell, or any other part our body.

If lack of sufficient oxygen is combined with a bad diet, pollutants, toxins in your environment, lack of sufficient vitamins, minerals, amino acids, and enzymes; the already weakened area, due to lack of oxygen, can go over the edge resulting in catastrophic failure of the most affected area of the body. Surgery and prescription drugs may take care of an immediate health crisis, but often are a temporary fix for a worsening overall health failure as declining health increasingly cascades downward.

Disease, bodily malfunctions, and organ failures happen most often where the body has been most weakened. Lack of oxygen severely and cumulative weakens our cellular body.

The reasons why we do not receive sufficient oxygen is a long list; just as the list of toxins and contaminants in our lives is very long:

- Pollution
- Cars and motor exhaust
- Perfumes and cleaning chemicals
- Declining levels of oxygen in air
- Synthetic clothing that does not allow skin to breathe
- Closed and sealed houses and buildings
- Paints and solvents

- Fuels and petroleum products
- Gas burning stoves and heating units in sealed buildings.
- Coal and gas burning power plants
- Synthetic fabrics that release chemical gases.
- Junk foods
- Artificial chemicals in food.
- Commercially farmed meat and vegetables.
- Processed foods.

The list is almost endless. The declining level of oxygen in our air is being replaced with massive amount of toxins and irritants. When starved of oxygen and devoid of essential nutrients, our cellular body can only take so much abuse. Once the threshold of what our body can expel or handle has been reached a health crisis is entirely predictable. Unfortunately, as we age such neglect, abuse, and damage accumulated; with remedy for these afflictions increasingly becoming an uphill climb.

We live in a society that glories doing whatever you want while assuming there are no consequences; to recklessly live for today as tomorrow will take care of itself. This is what we have been taught and conditioned to live by. But in reality it is tomorrow that you pay for the price of abuses today. People have become so comfortable and there is such an abundance of commercial advertising advocating harmful living and harmful products that it has become the social behavior norm.

The justification is that if everyone else lives this way then certainly it must be safe. That is the lemmings running over the cliff way of thinking. All of us see the growing health crisis all around us including so many people we personally know.

We are conditioned to think that when the inevitable illness and health failure comes, a person just has to go to the doctor for a prescription, surgery or therapy and health will quickly be restored – at astronomical costs.

In fact, while the immediate health crisis may be addressed, the underlying problem has not been cured because the source of the lack of wellness remains.

Why only treat symptoms while ignoring the problem?

We assume everything is just fine because everyone else lives like we do and they seem to be doing just fine. Advertisements and movies all show us what makes a person happy and healthy, right? We disregard the illness, disease, and sickness that we see all around us. We assume that we cannot get cancer, that Alzheimer's only affects other people, that COPD will never affect me or I will not have a heart attack – and then it happens.

Some people take a totally apathetic view that they will enjoyy life however they want and then accept whatever comes. That is easily said until the crisis really comes, and then the person is asking "Why me?" Most will then decide their only hope against all odds in hoping that a doctor has a magic pill, drug therapy or a quick fix surgery.

> *"Take care of your body. It is the only place you have to live."* Anonymous

Why is it that we refuse to believe our health, our life, needs care and maintenance foremost is up to each of us?

This book focuses on the wellness power of hydrogen peroxide. But hydrogen peroxide is not an isolated subject nor the single magic bullet. Rather, there must be full balancing of the fundamentals of good essential nutrients, cellular and health protection, how to best avoid health issues, how to address those you have, and how to maximize your physical and mental health all must be collectively applied.

What some people rarely realize is how much declining health – even if unknown – also negatively affects a person mentally; psychologically and in relation to other people. There is no rule of nature that states that as people age they must move slower, become increasingly resistant to physical activity, gain more and more weight, have worsening memory and mental focus. Changing emotions and mental abilities may be caused by declining physical health or failing cellular body chemistry.

Most of the greatest minds in history were elderly.

Curiously, older generations better understood many of the principles of the importance of oxygen. Many are quite simple. For example, urging that you sleep with a window open for fresh air. Advises Spring cleaning to clean everything in the house to remove the dust (most of which is not dust, but instead is dead skin, virus, bacteria, fungus, the feces of those creatures and mites.) They understood the benefits of a healthy meal. Previous generations understood the value of airing out the house and Spring cleaning.

Now we are told to seal every crack in a house to save electricity. But as you breathe and use the oxygen, how is it supposed to be replaced? This is why you sleep poorly, wake up coughing, often exhausted and not feeling fully refreshed as nature intends. Did the oxygen level drop to 17%? 15%? 12%? 10% during the night? How high did the carbon dioxide and carbon monoxide levels go up as you slept while the oxygen level increasingly went down?

It is known you need oxygen more than any other substance. Yet our modern way of living increasingly reduces how much we oxygen receive.

We know our bodies need vitamins, minerals, amino acids and enzymes. But we rarely ask if those are in our food. They no longer are in our diets or in our fruits and vegetables.

We know that most chemicals, toxins, and noxious odors are harmful. Yet we continue to consume chemicals, surround ourselves with chemicals, and use chemical. We drink, eat and swim in known dangerous chemicals when there are natural and even beneficial alternatives.

Why would anyone be surprised when their body starts giving out after years and decades of denial, neglect and abuse?

If you understand and practice the natural principles of cellular health and total wellness you will be amazed that not only will your physical health and energy levels will go up, but so will your level of joy and confidence. You may be surprised at how easy it is to do.

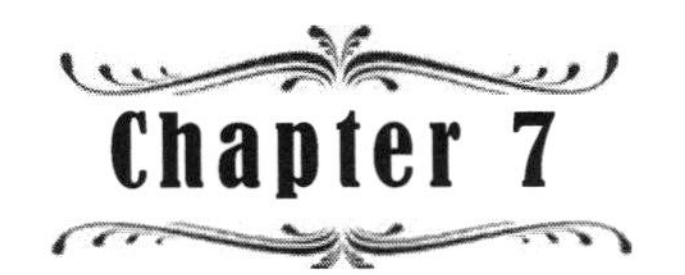

Chapter 7

Hydrogen Peroxide Protects & Restores Wellness

Oxygenation and oxygen therapies both protect and restores a person's wellness level, plus addresses both minor and major ailments and diseases.

Many people tend to avoid the word "cure" not only for regulatory and legal reasons, but also because health is so complex. With so many factors at play promising a "cure" is dubious and probably reckless.

No one else can legitimately "cure" either an injury or illness. Often there is no drug or surgery that will do so either. In nearly all instances, it is your own body that is providing the final cure. You and health professionals are only assisting your cellular body to do so.

Medical researchers across the world have found that many degenerative diseases are anaerobic. That means lacking oxygen. Degenerative disease cells usually cannot survive in an oxygen rich environment. Being anaerobic they cannot reproduce in oxygen and many tumors will literally build up a fluid barrier to try to block oxygen because oxygen will destroy it. Some tumors obtain their energy by fermenting sugar (glucose) rather than "burning" oxygen, a reason it is advisable to reduce sugar intake in certain health situations.

> "Deprive a cell 35% of its oxygen for 48 hours and it will become cancerous." Nobel Prize winner Otto Warburg of Germany made it clear that the root cause of cancer is oxygen deficiency, which creates an acidic state in the human body. Dr. Warberg discovered that cancer cells are anaerobic (do not use oxygen) and cannot survive in the presence of high levels of oxygen.

Healthy cells need oxygen. As stated, many tumor cells cannot survive in oxygen. Nobel Peace Prize Winner Otto Warburg of Germany, an early and respected researcher into oxygenation, claimed back in 1966 that when cells are receiving sufficient oxygen, tumor cells cannot exist.

Many degenerative diseases can be traced back to oxygen deprivation and poor cellular nutrition. Other health abuses hasten the development of such degenerative diseases and health failure.

Minerals are critical to cellular health and to optimize processing and utilization of oxygen – regardless of how your body is obtaining it – which is why later in this book minerals are so strongly suggested in your health supplemental nutritional personal protocol. A deficiency of essential minerals will minimize detoxification and oxygen usage and dispersal within the cellular body and blood stream.

How to get more oxygen into the body? There are many ways to do so.

Oxygen enters the body in 3 ways:

- Lungs
- Skin
- Digestive tract

Oxygen and essential nutrients through our skin

Most people believe we only gain oxygen through breathing. This is false. Certainly our lungs are critical and the intake of oxygen is their foremost function. Most oxygen a person receives is through the lungs. However this is not the only way.

Your skin breathes. It inhales and exhales. Healthy skin excretes toxins. It absorbs minerals and it absorbs oxygen. This is a reason to take care of your skin, avoid oils that block it, and to keep it clean of contaminates, bacteria, fungus, and mites as much as possible. Skin is not a layer of plastic wrap covering our bodies. If you wrap a person's skin entirely in plastic that person will die. After the James Bond movie Goldfinger, a woman sprayed her whole body with gold spray paint. She died as a result. Skin both being able to breathe and expel waste and toxins is critical.

This is the primary reason you need to exercise caution to prevent harmful. chemicals on your skin. This is particularly true of chlorine, ammonia, cleaning products, pesticides, gasoline, petroleum products, and oil based paints and thinners. To decide what to allow on your skin, ask yourself a simple question: "Would I drink this?" If not, you probably do not want it on your skin because your skin will absorb it.

This also is a reason to avoid tightly woven synthetic clothing and to minimize synthetic clothing. Natural clothing feels better against your skin, doesn't it? This is your body communicating to you. Synthetic clothing often also is leaching off chemicals and gags your skin of oxygen, similar to the way putting such material over your nose and mouth will restrict your breathing.

Oxygen and essential nutrients through our food and stomach

Do you know we receive oxygen through our food? More importantly food can be a major source of some (but not all) essential cellular nutrients. Most nutrients are destroyed when food is cooked. Vitamins such as C and B6 are totally destroyed by boiling. Boiling leaches out nearly all nutrients in food.

Cooking vegetables and fruits also destroys essential enzymes and amino acids. Beneficial nutrients in some cheeses are destroyed by heat. Cooking vegetables and fruits also eliminates nearly all oxygen in them.

High temperature cooking, frying and broiling alters natural fats found in meats, which converts the fat into a form that no longer has proper nutritional value. Instead, the meat becomes a substance that blocks the digestive system preventing absorption of both oxygen and nutrients. The overheated fat leads to plaque that lines the digestive system. It can cause blockage of the blood stream that not only prevents the blood transporting essential nutrients, but also can lead to stroke, heart attack and weakened vital organs.

Turn down your ovens when cooking to below 300 degrees for meat and vegetables. Be certain to still cook meat long enough for safety.

In the distant past, most meats were slow, low-temperature smoked or even sun dried after sea salted (sea salt is mineral rich.) Using low temperature cooking avoided destroying the meat's essential nutrients – and generally is far more tasty. They did not have the fatty taste because the fat had not been converted to a form similar to rancid lard.

Industry has made it very convenient to cook our food in ways that eliminates most of the food value and may cause it to become harmful; leaving only raw calories, starch, sugar, and little else other than what is harmful rather than beneficial. Yes, microwave ovens are very convenient. But they destroy virtually all nutritional value of food in terms of essential vitamins, minerals, amino acids, and necessary enzymes – while converting fats to a harmful form.

Our skin and digestive system both absorb oxygen and essential nutrients, expel toxins and waste materials, flush the body of dead cells and defeated bacteria, viruses, fungus and their waste excretions.

Lungs intake and expel oxygen and toxins

Our lungs are the great oxygen pumps of our body. But they also pump out harmful gases, specifically including carbon monoxide, as well as others. These problems are continually worsening. Humanity's lungs are under assault like never before. In the past, the oxygen level in atmosphere was significantly higher than now and the air was pure.

On average, the level of oxygen in the air is down to only 19% to 21% if in clean rural country air. This is lower than our bodies are meant to have due to declining percentage of oxygen in the atmosphere. If you live in an urban environment, the oxygen level in the air is even lower. In highly dense and enclosed urban spaces it can drop as low as 10%.

Usually such settings also mean the air is laced with a potent collection of toxins, pathogens, carbon monoxide and toxic and carcinogenic gases. This encourages shallow breathing further reducing our oxygen intake. Collectively this also causes a person's physical activities to decline, which hastens declining health, aging and weakening vital organs such as heart and lungs.

For energy efficiency, our homes and places of work are sealed, blocking air flow and sealing in rising air content of chemicals, dust (dead cells, bacteria, fungus, and their wastes), toxins, pesticides, and chemicals.

As a person ages in such an environment - always deficient of oxygen and essential cellular nutrients - is it any surprise that people's health can rapidly decline with age or suddenly collapse? Our cells and vital organs can only withstand oxygen and nutritional deprivation plus being increasingly bombarded by toxins, pathogens, and chemicals – and resulting little physical activity - for so long.

It is unlikely a prescription or surgery is going to put you back into whole wellness, is it? As our health declines, so does our mental focus, memory, eye sight, sense of taste, and hearing. Even mental health and positive psychology all take a terrible toll.

We become easily exhausted if low on oxygen lacking the motivation and energy of our youth. Step-by-step we start to give up without realizing what is happening. The physical and mental vigor and drive of our youth vanishes as our cellular body is weakened and deteriorates.

Until the arrival of antibiotics, physicians were advocating using hydrogen peroxide plus fresh unpolluted air to treating diseases. Literally thousands of medical studies and treatises on hydrogen peroxide and oxygen therapy were written and published worldwide including by Nobel Prize winners and renounced biochemists.

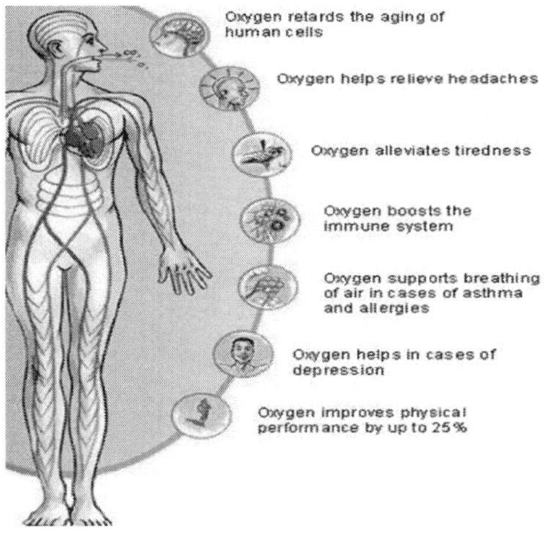

There is no vital nutrient that your cellular body needs more than oxygen. Hydrogen peroxide's working element is 100% pure oxygen.

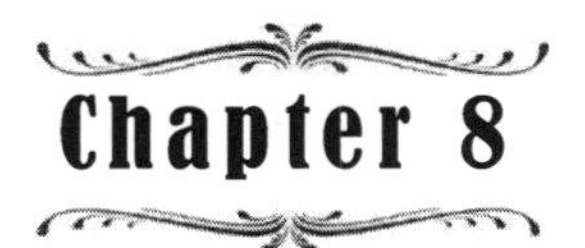

Chapter 8

Obesity On The Rise

> There is no diet that will do what eating healthy does. Skip the diet. Just eat healthy.

What is obesity on the rise? Because our cellular body is starving.

We eat so much and burn so few calories because we are starving. You can consume 2000, 3000, 4000, 7000 calories a day – yet you are starving. No matter how much you eat, your body subconsciously continues to scream: "EAT MORE! EAT MORE! EAT MORE!" Why?

People are becoming overweight because most people are starving at the cellular level, for which the cellular body makes the person feel constantly hungry.

What we do not consciously recognize is that your body is not starving for calories or hydrocarbons. It is starving for essential vitamins and trace minerals, amino acids, and enzymes – and for oxygen! So your body acts like you are starving, even if you are 10%, 40%, 100%, or 200% overweight. Your body can only hope you eat right and that you will give it oxygen.

Your cellular body does not know that now our food is devoid of nearly all essential minerals, amino acids and enzymes, with what little that remains generally destroyed in food processing and modern cooking. Our bodies are designed to rely upon food for minerals and nutrients. Therefore your inner-self, your cellular body, presumes that it will receive the additional nutrients you cells are lacking by constantly making you feel hungry.

Both junk food and healthy eating are addictive. Some processors of junk and processed foods add addictive substances to make you addicted to their food. So a greasy burger, french fries, friend chicken, or a taco from a fast foods place seemingly tastes good. Many people fool themselves into thinking that the little bit of lettuce, tomato, pickle and onion makes the food somehow healthy. Yet such food is less healthy than typical cheap cat and dog food.With a diet of junk foods, process foods, sugar or chemical sugar free sodas, we are literally eating ourselves to death – becoming obese while starving yourself to death of essential cellular nutrients.

A healthy diet and personal practice is also addictive. It takes about 30 days to wean off the addiction of junk food. Your body will love you for it. You will soon find you are not eating nearly as much. At first you will eat more because your cellular body wants more of those nutrients. However, soon you will eat less, because your body finally has the essential nutrients it needs. While organic and natural foods cost a little bit more to buy, in the long run they will cost you much less – particularly since you will not be driving through fast foods drive-thru lanes.

Within 90 days of a healthy diet, junk food will become repulsive to you. If you decide to have one of those big burgers on a bleached white bun and heavily table salted French fries you thought you used to enjoy - after one bite as that bad overheated fat and worthless bun hits your mouth -you will be repulsed by it. You also have reduced how many artificial chemicals you are consuming.

Your body knows what good food now is, and that horribly unhealthy and even harmful food will be subconsciously and consciously repulsive to you. A healthy diet is remarkably easy to follow and do.

The same will be true of corn syrup soda pop or chemical laced diet soda. It will come to taste horrible to you. You'll dump it out. If you reduce artificial colors and chemicals in your food, you would come to taste those chemicals and reject them. It takes about 30-90 days for that transition.

While you may think you don't have time to "cook," once you get in a habit of doing so is quick and enjoyable.

IF YOU WANT TO LOSE WEIGHT?

Do not start by counting calories. You are wasting your time.

- Make a list of the vitamin, mineral, amino acid and enzyme

- Buy easy but healthy organic and natural foods. If meat, buy fresh and organic. The same applies to fruits and vegetables.

- Throw away your table salt and use sea salts.

- Install a water filter on your kitchen faucet for your drinking water. Bottled water is not necessary. Such filters are inexpensive at hardware stores.

- Eliminate grocery store salt, and reduce white floor products, corn syrup products and processed sugar.

- Follow the oxygenation advice throughout this book.

- Use 35% food grade hydrogen peroxide oxygenation.

- Reduce chemical and toxicity in your home.

- Have a fresh air flow for your house and a small bedroom HEPA air filtration system.

- Wear natural materials clothing to the extent possible.

As you do the above eat all you want of your healthy food, while oxygenating your body and feeding your cells with all essential nutrients. Forget about counting calories and leave all the diet pills alone. Eat all you want of good, nutritious food as you otherwise feed your cells and body everything it needs.

Not only will you soon be eating less because you will not feel hungry, you will have increasing levels of energy – overtly and in metabolism. Your good healthy cells are running at full power. You are healthily burning calories. Your immune system is supercharged. Your organs are oxygen and nutrient rich. Your muscles are working the way they should. Your blood stream is a roadway of wellness.

Not only will you have levels of energy you have not had since your youth burning more calories, your mental and psychological outlook will change. Your complexion and skin will be enhanced. Internally, externally, and in outlook you are glowing.

You will be alert with better mental and psychological health. Your muscle aches and headaches will diminish or fade away. You will sleep better and it will be easier to get out of bed. Providing your cellular body the oxygen and nutrients it needs, while minimizing it being poised and handicapped by toxins and other harmful substances will product wondrous results.

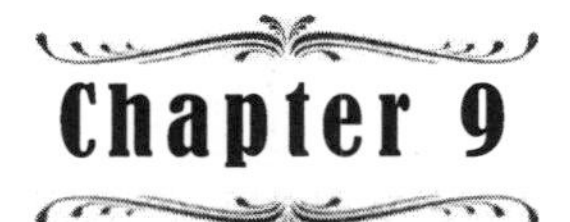

Chapter 9

Hydrogen Peroxide Oxygen Therapy

"The doctors of the future will give no medicine, but will interest the patient in the care of human frame, in the cause and prevention of disease, and in proper nutrition."

Thomas A. Edison

There are websites and books urging massive levels of oral intake of food grade hydrogen peroxide. You will not read this advice in this book. However, it does include present beneficial levels of oral intake of 35% food grade hydrogen peroxide as your cellular body directs you.

Elsewhere in this book, there also are additional ways to increase your oxygen intake for significant and unique benefits. Super-oxygenation also cleanses our cellular body of pathogens and harmful micro-organisms that 35% food grade hydrogen peroxide will destroy. This chapter specifically discusses hydrogen peroxide oxidation therapy.

1. Through your skin

Every other day, wipe 35% hydrogen peroxide that has been diluted to 2% and no more than 3% on your arms and legs. Do not use it any stronger. Only do so once, rather than keep wiping over and over. Do this in a shower. You may wish to add your stomach area. Remember that hydrogen peroxide can bleach clothing, hair and carpeting.

KEEP HYDROGEN PEROXIDE AWAY FROM YOUR EYES.

After wiping it on, wait a minute or two and wash it off by showering. Not only has your body absorbed much of the oxygen, you now have killed nearly all contaminating micro-organisms that are harmful and has removed most contaminants and dead skin cells clogging your skin's pores. Shower off before exiting the shower. Dry off with a cotton towel. If you wish to do so every day before you shower that is better still.

Hydrogen Peroxide may “bleach” (it is not really “bleaching”) color from clothing and your hair.

Also, twice a week take a soaking bath in comfortable water to which you have added 1.) hydrogen peroxide, 2.) sea salt (ideally Dead Sea Salt) and 3.) magnesium (Epson salt) available all drug stores.

Add 2 cups of 35% food grade hydrogen peroxide to your tub after you fill it. Add the sea salt (1-2 cups) and Epson salt (one-fourth to one-half pound) before so it can dissolve.

Remain in the tub for at least 15 minutes. Relax. If necessary add a little more hot water to keep the temperature comfortable. Then rinse off after the bath soak. If you want to do a brief wipe down with 2% to 3% hydrogen peroxide dilution before showing off, definitely do so.

Alternative method

Some people use a plastic spray bottle instead of a cloth for the food grade hydrogen peroxide. This is easier, faster and more complete. However, please wear safety goggles. You can buy those at any hardware store inexpensively. Hydrogen peroxide can be very damaging to the eyes very quickly. If using a spray bottle, safety goggles are a necessary safety precaution you should never neglect.

If you get hydrogen peroxide in your eyes immediately and repeatedly flush your eyes generously with water. Do not delay. You may want to have the shower running on very low so it is immediately available at a cool level just in case it gets in your eyes.

If you use a spray bottle, mark it as dangerous or as poison just in case a child or other person finds it and decides to play with it or sprays it on themselves or someone else for play including their eyes.

If children are in the home, always secure concentrated hydrogen peroxide under lock and key. Write on the bottle an appropriate warning if there are children or others in the house who need to be warned.

Through your Digestive System

This is controversial and is neither approved nor banned by the F.D.A. It is important to not be excessive. There are materials in circulation we believe discussing this topic. The decision, ultimately, is yours.

It is not possible to give a usage schedule identical for everyone, though many materials give exact levels of usages disregarding we are all unique.

- We are all different sizes and weight
- We have different rates metabolisms
- We each have different general health and wellness issues
- We are of different ages
- We each are breathing a different level of oxygen in air
- We have different diets
- We follow other different manners of oxygenation
- We take different nutritional supplements

The guidelines for each person varies because we are each unique – and so is each person's internal cellular body. In the following steps you personalize usage levels to your specific, personal correct level.

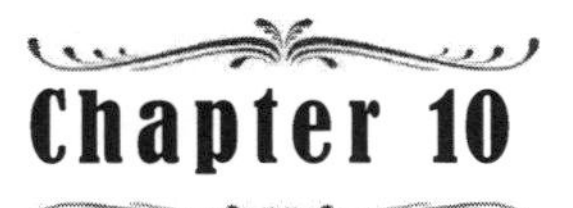

Chapter 10

Oral Super-Oxygenation

35% Food Grade Hydrogen Peroxide

(Subligual Hydrogen Peroxide Biotherpeutics)

1st Start slow. If you start too fast and with too many drops you may quickly discontinue following your personal protocol. It takes a while to acquire a taste for hydrogen peroxide. Your body has to adjust to it, as does the beneficial flora in your digestive system.

2nd Do not take hydrogen peroxide at meal time as you will develop a gassy stomach. The food also interferes with the absorption.

3rd Do not internally take hydrogen peroxide within 1 hour of taking any prescription medication as it can alter the prescription.

Week 1

4 drops of 35% Food Grade Hydrogen Peroxide

In 6 ounces distilled water* twice a day

***You may use juice if you prefer, but do not pre-mix juice in advance.**

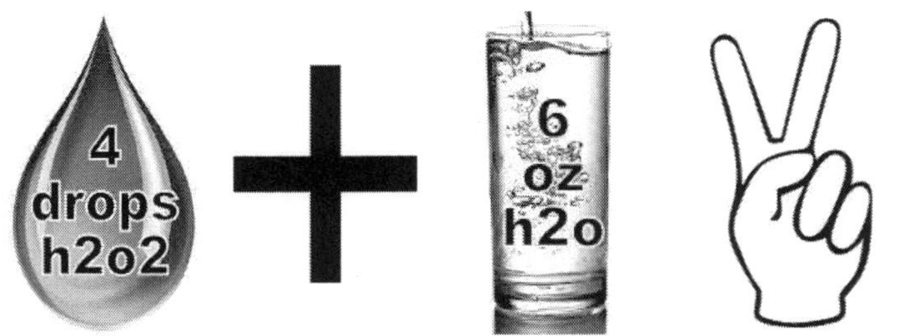

***Distilled water is ideal. But you may use juice if you prefer, but do not pre-mix juice in advance. This may help you become accustomed to the taste.**

Week #1: Start with twice a day. Midmorning or midafternoon and an hour or 2 after your evening meal is ideal. You may later wish to increase this to 3 times a day. Repeat this schedule daily for 6 days, skipping the 7th day.

Unless you in a severe medical health crisis circumstance for which you may decide to try starting at a higher level and advancing more quickly, start out at 4 drops of 35% food grade hydrogen peroxide in 6 ounces of distilled water or filtered water.

You may experience some level of diarrhea at first. This is your body flushing toxins – which is a good thing. That will not continue for long.

Give Your Body 1 Day Of Rest Each Week

> "...and on the seventh day God ended his work which he had made; and he rested..." Genesis 2:2

Always skip the 7th day. This is advisable for all supplements you take. This allows your body to rest and to balance out any excesses you may be developing. This applies to all dietary and health supplements except any prescription medication you are taking. Do not skip prescriptions.

Week 2

8 drops of 35% Food Grade Hydrogen Peroxide

In 8 ounces distilled water* three times a day

Increase by 1 to 2 drops per week

***You may use juice if you prefer, but do not pre-mix juice in advance.**

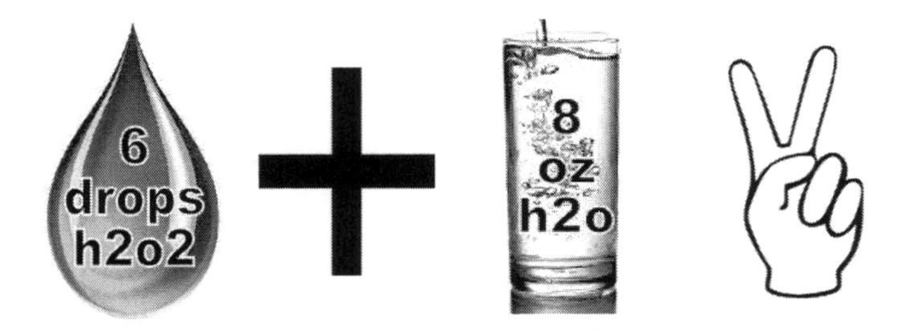

For week #2: Increase to 8 drops. If you wish a higher level, increase to 3 times a day: midmorning, midafternoon and midevening. Again, skip the 7th day. If you miss a day, do not use double the next time.

If you feel comfortable with doing so, for week three you may increase to 8 drops in 8 ounces of water, 2 to 3 times a day.

Week 3 & Thereafter

7 drops of 35% Food Grade Hydrogen Peroxide
In 6 ounces distilled water* 2 or 3 times a day

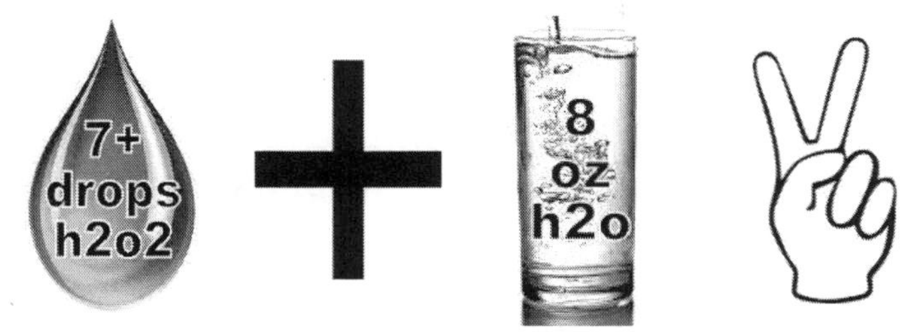

***You may use juice if you prefer, but do not pre-mix juice in advance.**

Week #3 and thereafter: You may increase this by 1 to 2 more drops in 8 ounces of distilled or filtered water 2 or 3 times a day as each week passes as you feel comfortable with.

How Much To Increase The Number of Drops?

Increase as you feel comfortable. Try 3 times a day and continue to increase, but not at an uncomfortable rate. If you are battling a serious condition and have opted to use hydrogen peroxide as part of your total protocol you may wish to increase at a faster rate. However, remember, more is not always better.

There are warning signs of excessive usage. If your eyes start becoming bloodshot looking you are over oxygenating or you are experiencing notable stomach discomfort, stop for 2 days and return at a lower level.

Upon reaching a High Level of Usage

Be very careful evolving past 20 drops at a time. Beyond that level will be too high for most people. Exercise caution before increasing to high mega-dosing. Excessive usage is counter-productive.

Remember, compared to other materials you may read, you are also oxygenating through your skin and mouth, which few other materials advise. It is more beneficial and effective to use hydrogen peroxide therapy on different areas of your body to do so – plus there are notable and real advantages to sterilizing your mouth and for doing so for large areas of your skin. Doing so directly oxygenating your skin, the largest organ of your body of many vital functions.

We are each unique and of different sizes, weights, ages, activity levels, diet and health. Your cellular body is guiding you to the correct level.

WARNINGS

If you are experiencing significant problems in ingesting hydrogen peroxide, cease doing so. Each person has different health challenges.

Never self-inject hydrogen peroxide directly into your body by needle injection or any other method of directly putting into your blood stream. The filtration system of your digestive system, mouth and skin is essential to being able to beneficially and safely use the oxygen. For intravenous hydrogen peroxide you must have this done by fully qualified doctor or healthcare professional.

Worse, you may cause massive and permanent injury putting hydrogen peroxide directly into your blood stream. This cannot be too stressed. You destroy your health permanently if you attempt to do so.

Intravenous hydrogen peroxide is not done with food grade hydrogen peroxide. It has to be done at a specific rate, with specific dilution and in specific manners. People have been seriously and permanently injured attempting to personally inject hydrogen peroxide intravenously. There are licensed medical doctors and health practitioners who offer intravenous hydrogen peroxide treatment.

If you are facing a current medical health crisis or if you are perpetually ill with cold and flu type symptoms, I would highly suggest you seek out a licensed medical doctor to discuss intravenous hydrogen peroxide therapy to kick-start super-oxygenation and purification therapy.

Caution about wrong usage of hydrogen peroxide

Unfortunately, there is a lot of dangerous advice on the Internet and some has been repeated by so many that it seems legitimate. Doing what is listed below on this page (1-3) is never safe and may be harmful in permanent ways.

1. Never hydrogen peroxide in your eyes regardless of the concentration level. If you get hydrogen peroxide in your eyes, immediately flush your eyes with water (or any other drinkable liquid).

2. Never put concentrated hydrogen peroxide in your ears. This can permanently damage your ear drums.

3. Never spray hydrogen peroxide into your lungs by a nebulizer unless this is supervised by a qualified doctor or other qualified healthcare professional.

You have to decide whether you wish to use hydrogen peroxide for health and wellness. I have personally taken hydrogen peroxide orally for decades. If I did not fully believe it beneficial to me, I would not have continued to do so. Nor would other people do so that I know. I have never known anyone harmed by hydrogen peroxide super-oxygenation as described because we follow the safety rules. I know many who claim many profound positive effects. You have to decide for yourself.

I also have personally had hydrogen peroxide biotherapeutic oxygenation intravenously on numerous occasions and know others who have. Without exception, this was done by a licensed medical doctor at the doctor's facility. If you are in a severely medical situation with a degenerative disease, cancer, are continually ill by colds, flu or infections, you may wish to seek a qualified medical profession to jump-start hydrogen peroxide based super-oxygenation intravenously.

How to find a qualified medical doctor or healthcare professional for intravenous hydrogen peroxide therapy?

First, search the Internet. It is an excellent resource. If you have difficulty finding this service offered, you may have better results by searching for a qualified healthcare professional who does "chelation." Chelation is not that same procedure, but most professionals who do chelation also will do intravenous hydrogen peroxide treatments.

What is Chelation Therapy?

Just for your information, chelation is an intravenous process used to extract harmful heavy metals from the body. If you opt to have chelation, it is very important to understand that chelation extracts vital minerals from the body along with the harmful heavy metals, leaving your body severely depleted of essential minerals. After a chelation treatment it is vital that a person immediately take a large quantity of all minerals including all trace minerals.

Hydrogen Peroxide super-oxygenation is not a stand-alone solution.

It is critical to remember that hydrogen peroxide cellular oxidation therapy is only one part of a greater protocol:

- Increasing oxygen to your blood, including as simple as fresh air for your home and the many other ways.

- Providing the other essential nutrients your cells, organs and brain need.

- Eliminating toxins, pathogens, harmful chemicals and bad food as much as possible.

However, you should also:

- Maximize oxygen intake in the air that you breathe.

- Minimize chemicals, toxins and pathogens entering your body through the air you breathe, food you eat and what comes into contact with your skin.

- Insure that your cellular body has all the needed vitamins, minerals and amino acids.

You do not have to follow any of these guidelines perfectly. Do not guilt-trip if you forget now and then, or even fall off the wagon for a while. Do not double up next time. Return to your protocol and continue with the level of progression that you had reached.

Chapter 11

How To Reduce Hydrogen Peroxide Concentration

This chapter explains how to reduce the concentration of 35% food grade hydrogen peroxide if you develop a specific usage reason to do so.

Use 35% food grade hydrogen peroxide (see Chapter 4 discussion of why only use 35%).

Reducing the concentration of 35% food grade hydrogen peroxide is simple mathematics.

35% means it is 35% concentrated – the highest concentration legal to sell to consumers and ship. It also is the only concentration of "food grade" that is consumer available.

Reducing to 3%

To make 3% hydrogen peroxide, mix 1 parts of 35% food grade hydrogen peroxide to 11 part of distilled or filtered water.

Reducing to 8%

To make 8%, mix 1 parts of 35% food grade hydrogen peroxide to 4 part of distilled or filtered water.

Reducing to 17.5%

To make 17.5%, mix 1 parts 35% food grade hydrogen peroxide to 1 part distilled of filtered water.

Reducingto other ratios percentage levels

For other dilution ratios just do the math. For internal usage, you must greatly reduce the concentration. See Chapter 10 above on Hydrogen Peroxide therapy.

PRE-MIXING:

Some people prefer to dilute 35% for convenience and safety reasons prior to storage. Use a clean plastic container, use only distilled water and mark it as dangerous. Write the date on the container.

Store it in a cool, dark location. Secure hydrogen peroxide if children are in the home. Use a highlighter to mark the concentration you reduced it to and add warnings for others.

If you pre-mix or pre-dilute hydrogen peroxide for later, use distilled water. For safety reasons, do not use a glass container. Mark the bottle with a poison symbol or other manner so no one accidently drinks it in concentrated from.

*Ideally use distilled water with hydrogen peroxide. However, if you are using juices, spring water, or well water, do not pre-mix more than 1 hour before usage as certain elements in those liquids will break down the hydrogen peroxide reducing its strength.

UV light breaks down hydrogen peroxide. Store hydrogen in the dark and away from a heat source.

Wear gloves and goggles while mixing and pouring if concentrated.

If you spill hydrogen peroxide on your skin just wash it off. There may be temporary skin bleaching and stinging of your skin. No permanent damage has been done. Color will return and stinging will stop generally in 15 to 30 minutes. Remember that there are no toxins that can be absorbed.

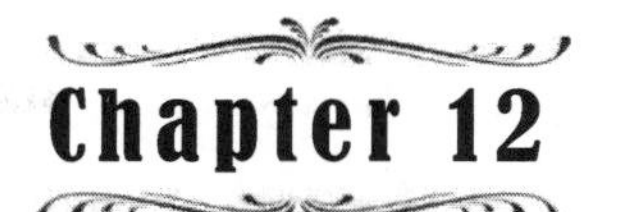

Chapter 12

Essential Cellular & Body Support

Many people seeking natural and alternative health maintenance and those wishing to address health issues can become so lost in all the promises in herbal, homeopathic, mega-dosing vitamins or other supplements, or other promises, they forget the essential basics.

It is worthwhile to list what are the most essential necessities of your cells, body and vital organs:

VITAMINS

While you can obtain the vitamins in your food, few people consistently eat a diverse enough diet to do so sufficiently.

You do not need to buy extremely expensive or exotic vitamin pills. You will want about 200% - 300% the USDA recommended minimal daily level, depending on your weight, metabolism and quality of your diet. Do not take radically high level of vitamins.

CALCIUM

Calcium is also critical to good health for many reasons. It is important to understand the body cannot process calcium without both magnesium and Vitamin D. Most people avoid a large amount of sunlight which causes a Vitamin D deficiency. The benefits of magnesium are enormous and the damages of a magnesium deficiency are severe.
See chapter 17 on Magnesium.

Do not take extreme levels of calcium supplementing. Doing so can cause kidney and gallstones. Depending on your weight and whether you intake calcium in other ways, try approximately 200% to 300% of the USDA's recommended daily recommended level, but no higher.

You can find calcium supplements that also contain magnesium and Vitamin D. If you receive a lot of sunlight on your skin you can use less vitamin D but still must supplement with magnesium. However, excessive radiation from direct intense sunlight is harmful.

MAGNESIUM

In the chapter on magnesium, the critical importance of magnesium is explained and documented by legitimate research and medical studies from around the world. You can take magnesium orally and through the skin. This is discussed extensively in Chapter 17.

TRACE MINERALS

Our food today is seriously deficient in trace minerals regardless of how natural you make your diet. Trace minerals are essential nutrients for your cellular and vital organs' health. Start your personal wellness protocol with a moderately high level to restore essential trace minerals your cells have probably been lacking for a long time.

A good liquid mineral supplement with a weekly bath soak described in this book with 35% food grade hydrogen peroxide, sea salt and magnesium (Epson's Salt) will meet this essential need.

AMINO ACIDS

Like trace minerals, amino acids also are an essential cellular nutrient. Take an amino acid supplement. Start with a moderately high level.

PROBIOTICS

Probiotics are beneficial micro-organisms necessary for food and stomach processing. A probiotic supplement is highly advised to insure your digestive system is properly functioning.

HYALURONIC ACID

Hyaluronic acid is the lubricant between skeletal joints. As a person ages their body produces less of it. This generally means joint pain and stiffness. This may lead to joint and nerve damage. If you are past 40 or highly active, taking hyaluronic acid supplementing will avoid and address joint pain and damage often with astonishing benefits.

B12 AND B VITAMINS

B12 and B vitamins are important to the nervous system and metabolic process. They also are beneficial to mental health.

Never take B vitamins by pill. They are not absorbed through the stomach. Use a liquid B12 complex under your tongue (called "sublingual") or a dissolvable tablet under the tongue. Do not chew it.

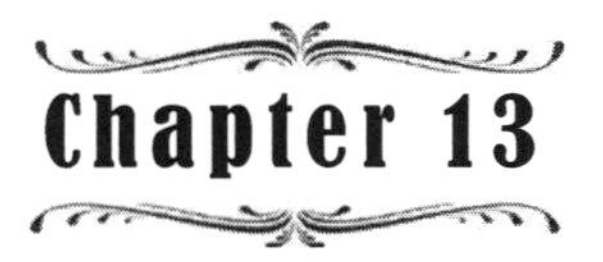

Chapter 13

Removing Toxins From Your Home: Chlorine

> The competent physician, before he attempts to give medicine to the patient, makes himself acquainted not only with the disease, but also with the habits and constitution of the sick man." Cicero

Are you filling your air with deadly gases? Do you bathe in highly toxic chemicals?

The two most common pool and spa chemicals are chlorine and bromine.

Did you know those are two of the most deadly chemicals on earth?

.

Known Chlorine Dangers

- Chlorine combines with natural organic matter decaying vegetation to form potent cancer causing trihalo methanes (THM's)
- Chlorine joins with other substances to make carcinogens as chloroforms, bromoforms carbon tectachloride, bischlorothane and other cancer causing agents
- The level of chlorine in swimming pools is over 1,000% the level deemed minimally safe by the EPA in water
- Causes atherosclerosis, stroke and heart attack
- Causes skin to prematurely age
- Damages the human eye

- Causes bladder, breast, testicular, colon, rectal and bowel cancer, and malignant melanoma

- Damages lung tissue

- Causes acne, psoriasis, seborrhea and eczema

- Converts to dioxins – among the most dangerous of cancer causing chemicals, which build up permanently within a person's body. Dioxins also cause infertility and birth defects

- Damages the nervous system permanently

"Chlorine is so dangerous" according to PhD biologist/chemist Dr. Herbert Schwartz "that it should be banned. Putting chlorine in water is like starting a time bomb. Cancer, heart trouble, premature senility, both mental and physical are conditions attributable to chlorine treated water supplies. It is making us grow old before our time by producing symptoms of aging such as hardening of the arteries."

Dr. Stephen Askin wrote: "The real issue is not just how toxic chlorine itself is but how the unintended by-products of chlorine (organochlorines and dioxins) remain in the environment. They are persistent in the environment; they do not break down readily and therefore bio-accumulate. This can create a very serious health problem; the dioxins and other toxic chemicals accumulate in the fatty tissues. These contaminants are also hormone disrupters because they mimic estrogen."

The U.S. Environmental Protection Agency (EPA) has observed and documented hormonal imbalance, suppressed immune systems, reproductive infertility, and alterations in fetal development of animals. In viewing the big picture these factors are perhaps the most frightening results from the widespread use of chlorine.

In Super Nutrition for Healthy Hearts, ***Dr. Richard Passwater*** shows how ***"the origin of heart disease is akin to the origin of cancer"*** Chlorination could very well be a key factor linking these two major diseases. Chlorine creates THM's and haloforms. These toxic chemical can trigger the production of excess free radicals in our bodies. Free pollutants radicals cause cell damage. Excess free radicals can cause normal smooth muscle cells in the arterial wall to go haywire and to mutate to tumor cells. The fibrous plaque consequently formed is essentially a benign tumor. Unfortunately, this tumor is linked with the origin of heart disease."

Is Bromine a safe alternative? No.

Known Bromine Dangers:

- If spilled on skin it produces painful sores
- Has strong unpleasant odor
- Is Toxic
- Converts to dichlorobromomethane, bromoform and bromate

The Metropolitan Emergency Response Network defines the resulting dichlorobromomethan as particularly dangerous and harmful (see below). The vapors damage the eyes and lungs

- Causes cancer
- Damages skin
- Damages the liver
- Causes depressionn and brain damage
- Damages the nervous system and muscles
- Bromine vapors are known to reduce male sperm count and cause malformed DNA and chromosomes resulting in birth defects and causes male infertility
- Maximum safety precautions should be used when handling it

The Metropolitan Emergency Response Network manual clearly advises:

"Dichlorobromomethane should be handled as a CARCINOGEN--WITH EXTREME CAUTION.* Exposure can irritate the eyes, nose and throat. Higher levels can irritate the lungs and may cause you to become dizzy, light-headed and to pass out. Could cause death. * Repeated exposures affect the liver. * Contact can irritate the skin."

WORSE, some pool and spa suppliers urge using both chlorine and bromine together - which doubles their sales. **Combining chlorine and bromine may be the second most powerful cancer-causing liquid mixture only surpassed by drinking highly radioactive liquids.**

DANGERS OF COMBINING CHLORINE AND BROMINE

When combined, chlorine and bromine make 97 carcinogens, 82 mutagens, 28 acute and chronic toxic contaminants, and 23 tumor promoters. Many complex chemicals result from the conversion of chlorine and bromine to poise other even more health devastating chemicals permanently accumulate in a person's body fat.

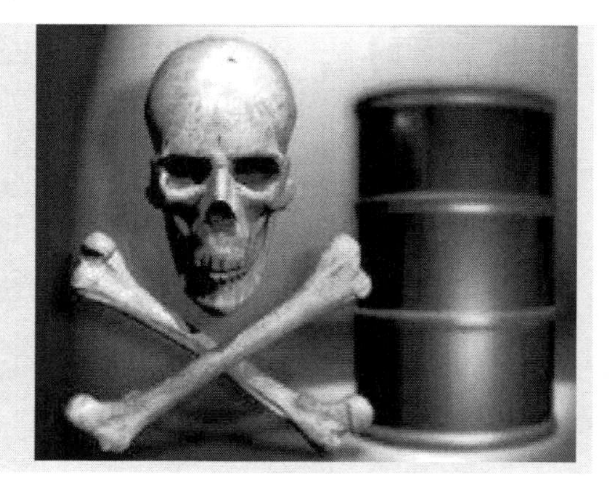

Each time a person is exposed, the level of carcinogens, mutagens, toxins, and tumor promoters increase. With each increase, the risk of cancer increases to a point it no longer being a question of whether or not the person will develop cancer. It is only a question of how soon. Each exposure to the chemicals from that point determines sooner or later.

To dive into a swimming pool and claim "See? I wasn't harmed" would be no different than a person holding up radioactive material, drinking it, and making the same claim. Both cause carcinogens and health damaging elements to house within the person's body – primarily in body fat. The more frequently the exposure the higher the level becomes.

Who makes such a claim that chlorine and bromine are dangerous and destructive to a person's health? Essentially every chemist, doctors in the field of environmental toxins, the EPA, medical researchers, and essentially all health professionals and experts in the fields of cancer and toxins, except those employed by the chemical manufacturers of chlorine and bromine. Chlorine also is the number one cause of household poisoning and is particularly dangerous to children.

> In 1997, 217,989 calls were made to the Poison Control Center. Of those calls, 62,023 were about chlorine. So, that means that 28.4% of all Poison Control Center calls were related to poisonings by chlorine products. What is even more important, most of those calls were about children under 6 years old.

The difference between chlorine and bromine compared to hydrogen peroxide is clear. Chlorine and bromine are two of the most deadly poisons in existence, both in immediate lethality and long term lethality on the DNA and cellular systems.

Oxygen is not toxic. Nor is water. Hydrogen peroxide is water and oxygen, the two most essential and beneficial elements to human life. The contrast is between the two of the most deadly chemicals on earth (chlorine and bromine) that also form even more horrifically known harmful chemicals to one of the most beneficial (hydrogen peroxide) is decisive and clear.

PROTECT YOUR CHILDREN AND GRANDCHILDREN

The health damages of chlorine and bromine are cumulative. The younger the person, the more likely they will develop serious, permanent or fatal disease, birth defects of their own children, and the other extremely harmful health effects. Compounding this is that young children tend to swallow more water in a swimming pool and spa.

Even if you foolishly decide that filling your body with permanent toxins and dioxins by swimming it those chemicals in your pool or spa is a risk you will continue to take or is not worth the bother to avoid, it is unthinkable to expose children to swimming in such water with the long term devastating health damage well known.

HOW DANGEROUS IS CHLORINE?

One recent study revealed that a non-smoker with a chlorinated pool is over twice as likely to develop cancer as a heavy smoker without a pool.

The high number of pools and spas using chlorine in the United States may well be the reason that cancer rates in deaths in the United States generally are 200% to 600% higher many than other countries, with similar differences in many other degenerative diseases. Millions Americans are unknowingly putting exorbitantly dangerous chemicals that are the top 10 most deadly toxins and carcinogens in the world into their pools and hot tubs - and then swimming in it and breathing the fumes.

VAPOR DANGERS:

The dangers of chlorine and bromine are not only within the water, but far worse health damage is caused by the moist vapors constantly in the air from the chemically laced water. The air from such a pool or spa subjects those around it and the household near it to continuously breathing high concentrations of such a damaging chemical mixture. The harmful vapors surrounding a chlorine and bromine treated pool or spa makes it a continual source of escalating health damage.

PERSONAL HEALTH:

It is amazing to see people drinking$1 bottles of water to avoid tap water, while sitting beside chlorine and bromine treated swimming pool or spa. A swim in that pool equals more than 1 year of drinking chlorinated water and is a devastatingly deadly soup of harmful toxins and carcinogens.

Chlorine and bromine, and the other deadly chemicals they combine with and make, that you intake into your body by your lungs and skin contact is literally engaging in self-executed chemical warfare against the cells of your cellular body. Nor do I exaggerate. Chlorine gas was the most lethal chemical used for chemical warfare in World War 1. Chlorine is extremely destructive to your cells. It causes D.N.A. damage to your cells, the primary cause of cancer, and disables cellular functionality.

Starves your body's cells. Poisons them. Attacks your blood vessels and is a chemical attack again against your nervous system. Burns your lungs oxygen sacks. It disrupts every organ in your body including your brain.

PRIORITIES AND THE ECONOMICS OF PERSONAL HEALTH

Good Health Equals True Wealth

Does using cheap pool and spa chemicals make economic sense? What is the cost of catastrophic health failure? Was the reason you bought your pool of spa to devastate your health and that of your family members and friends? Doing so is economically foolish. But the other reason to use hydrogen peroxide in your pool and spa is because now you avoid using your pool or spa due to the chemicals and their smell. The fumes and chemical drive you away from using your pool or spa.

Why people switch to 35% food grade hydrogen peroxide for their pools and spas:

Life is better by the pool

Wellness reasons are not the only reason people cease using chlorine and bromine in their pools, spas and hot tubs. Not everyone is health conscious.

Another reason is switch to hydrogen peroxide for your pool or spa to answer a simple question: Why do most people not use their pool or spa more than they do? How often does a person plan to use it, but then for some reason do not?

While many people switch for reasons of personal health, many have even another reason. They want to enjoy using their pool or spa. They do not want to smell their pool or spa chemicals. There is no smell if you use hydrogen peroxide instead. The main reason people with pools and spas quickly come to rarely actually use – or even sit by – their pool or spa is instinctive health repulsion to those deadly chemicals that your cellular body recognizes is harmful by the smell, even if you do not consciously recognize the danger. The water stings your eyes and turns them red. Skin turns white to deep layers. The chemicals severely harm your cells. Your cellular body tried every way to keep you out of and far away from the chemically laced water and air.

People familiar with 35% food grade hydrogen peroxide treatment of pools and spas will not use toxic pool chemicals. To no surpass, knowledgeable people do not want to relax or swim in toxic chemicals or breathe toxic fumes. Rather, they want to relax in pure, healthy, and clean water while breathing clean, fresh air.

It also is increasingly understood that pool chemicals interact with other chemicals and organics that enter a pool or spa, the chemical composition of the pool chemicals change to even more dangerous and harmful chemicals. The list is long and varies for different pool chemicals. Included are chemicals known to cause cancer and known to cause DNA corruption, lung, liver, brain damage and so many other health devastations. Those other formed chemicals are highly toxic complex molecular structures.

When any organic life form is destroyed, a result is the formation of ammonia. Most pool chemicals contain chlorine or bleach (or derivatives). Bleach and ammonia combined form chlorine gas, which also is what used in death penalty gas chambers and another WWI chemical weapon involving chlorine.

Those lethal chemicals continue to build up with each treatment by pool chemicals. Those chemicals also convert to other dangerous complex chemicals. Quickly, the pool becomes a toxic chemical trench, rather than the pure water swimming pond hoped for. The combination the toxins and chemicals would destroy a person's body within minutes if they were not diluted by the water in your pool. Instead, your health is steadily destroyed insidiously across time by damage to your cells.

Most people who switch to 35% food grade hydrogen peroxide for their pool or spa do so because they are health conscious. However, many also switch because their pool or spa is more enjoyable to use and be around for the lack of noxious fumes and because their subconscious natural defenses are not triggering a sense of warning and unpleasantness.

The Body's Natural-Defensives Smell Factor:

To understand the ***"smell"*** benefits of hydrogen peroxide over dirty water with organic wastes and the smell of chemicals in a treated pool or spa is to understand what hydrogen peroxide is and what it does in nature.

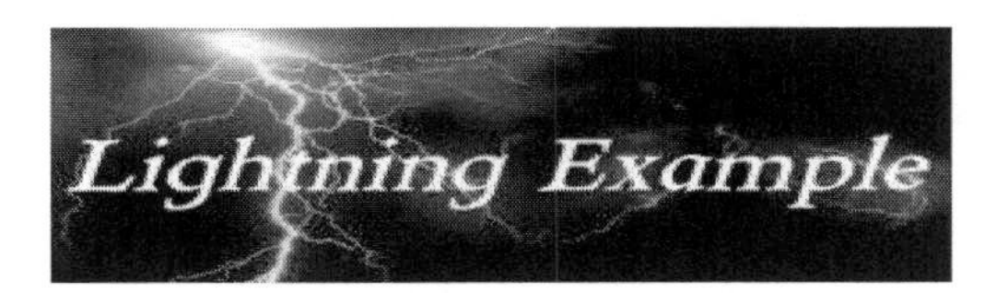

In nature, hydrogen peroxide appears only in trace amounts and only briefly. Hydrogen peroxide can be found in trace amounts sometimes in fast moving mountain streams.

Hydrogen peroxide is created in nature by lightning. During an electrical storm the air will come to have a crisp, fresh and clean smell to it. It is not just that the air is electrically charged, it also has increasing trace amounts of hydrogen peroxide that sterilizes the air and increases the oxygen level in the air.

Pure hydrogen peroxide will exist only briefly in nature. Hydrogen peroxide action is why the air seems so fresh. The air has been purified by the lightning and the hydrogen peroxide, which also eliminated many of bacteria, fungus and viruses in the air. The air will smell sweet, clean, somewhat damp and a bit heavy, although in an attractive way.

With the U.V. light from the clearing clouds or sunrise, the hydrogen peroxide decomposes to atoms of pure water vapor and pure gaseous oxygen. The air smells cleaner because it is cleaner, damp because of the pure water vapor in individual water atoms, and a bit heavy in an attractive way for the higher level of oxygen in the air. The water in a 35% food grade hydrogen peroxide treated pool or spa and the air around it is pleasing and desirable. Pure water and pure oxygen are beneficial to a person.

You may be wondering, "Isn't this book about the hydrogen peroxide? Why so much about other chemicals and issues such as chlorine?" The reason is because this book is about the path to true wellness in real, usable ways that you can easily follow and afford.

Being contrasted in this chapter are two different chemicals that exist both in liquid and gaseous form. Chlorine is one of the most deadly and health destructive substances on earth of devastating and worsening damage to your entire body. As it decomposes, it joins to other substances in nature to make an extensive list of health destroying complex chemical molecular strings. To the exact opposite, hydrogen peroxide is beneficial to your body – internally and externally. Your body even manufactures trace amounts of hydrogen peroxide if your cellular body has sufficient oxygen and essential nutrients.

Unlike Chlorine and bromine, when hydrogen peroxide decomposes it converts to only pure water and pure oxygen. There is nothing toxic or harmful in the simple and natural hydrogen peroxide structure which consists only of water and oxygen – 2 of the 4 essentials of life. .

Chlorine (which includes bleach) is one of the deadliest of all substances.

Hydrogen peroxide is one of the most beneficial.

Which one of those more comes in contact with and enters your body through your lungs, skin and stomach? The answer reveals a major reason why so many people are suffering from health failure, cancer and so many other degenerative diseases.

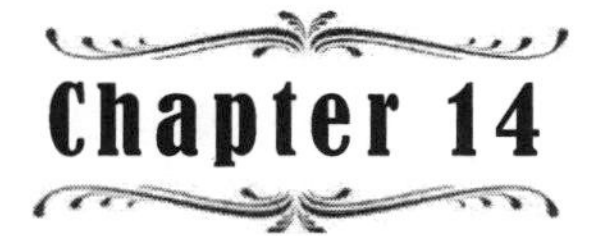

Chapter 14

Hydrogen Peroxide for Pool, Hot Tub & Spa

The previous Chapter 13 explains why you absolutely should eliminate chlorine and bromine from your pool, hot tub and spa.

> Imagine having a hot tub or pool that is odorless, will not harm anyone nor any plants or animals, and is highly beneficial to you? This is one of the many miracles of the power of hydrogen peroxide.

35% food grade hydrogen peroxide in pool treatment is not only non-toxic and not harmful. Instead, hydrogen peroxide is beneficial to your skin by oxygenating skin (rather than bleaching and poisoning it) and by cleansing your skin of organisms and contaminates, while removing dead skin.

As the elements of 35% food grade hydrogen peroxide are only pure water and pure oxygen, it will naturally decompose in its usage cycle of decomposition into pure and safe atoms of water and oxygen only. Thus, there is no chemical-build up; nor conversion to other chemical compositions. The fastest growing usage of 35% food grade hydrogen peroxide in the United States is for pools, hot tubs and spas.

Spa Usage and Costs

I cannot imagine anyone with a spa using any toxic and nauseous chemicals in their spa particular for the mist they make. The cost difference makes hydrogen peroxide attractive if all costs are figured. While 35% food grade hydrogen peroxide can cost more than some pool chemicals, if you add the numerous support chemicals, testing, and the price of the medical bills for the health damages for total cost comparison, 35% food grade hydrogen peroxide is a bargain.

If you try 35% food grade hydrogen peroxide in your spa, you will fall in love with your spa again and never go back to chlorine, bromine or secret ingredient pool chemicals. The 35% food grade hydrogen peroxide will eliminate the bad smells that come from untreated spa water and have none of the chemical smell of spa treatment chemicals. Every time you add chlorine and/or bromine to your pool or spa, you are increasing the level of one of the most deadly chemicals and toxins known to life.

Pond Maintenance

Hydrogen peroxide also can be used in ponds with plants to reduce algae and micro-organism growth.

The finest commercial aquariums now use 35% food grade hydrogen peroxide to treat their tanks, which contain fish and aquatic life inventories valued into the tens and hundreds of thousands of dollars. Draining and cleaning tanks is extremely costly, dangerous to sea life that has to be removed and particularly harmful to plant life that cannot be removed. However, they cannot use the toxic chemicals such as chlorine.

What they found is that 35% food grade hydrogen peroxide "attacks" the lowest life forms first – meaning the micro-organisms such as fungus and bacteria that harms their sea life. Next, the 35% food grade hydrogen peroxide will attack algae and lower plant life forms. They cease increasing the concentration of 35% food grade hydrogen peroxide treatment level at that point to avoid harm to the higher plant, fish and other aquatic life. The 35% food grade hydrogen peroxide that remains in the water will quickly decompose to merely pure water and gaseous oxygen by its interaction with the organic matter in the tank and U.V. from the display lights or sunlight if outdoors.

I do not recommend amateur usage of 35% food grade hydrogen peroxide in ponds or aquariums with fish. This requires fairly exact testing of concentration levels and supervision that is best left to the professionals in marine life. However, 35% food grade hydrogen peroxide treatment is an outstanding way to minimize algae, fungus and other infestations growth from turning a beautiful pond into a smelly, cloudy mini swamp.

SAFETY COMPARISON

Once hydrogen peroxide is diluted in your pool or spa at the correct level there are no safety issues. When diluted, all danger vanishes. 35%

food grade hydrogen peroxide contains no toxins or any harmful substance. It is water and oxygen. It does not cause cancer. It does not harm or age skin (it restores skin). It does not harm the liver, nervous system or brain. Hydrogen peroxide in your pool or spa as the water treatment will not and cannot harm you.

Once in the pool or spa, it is 100% safe, completely non-harmful and actually beneficial to your health to swim or soak in. No chemicals are needed to be added to your pool or spa. Just refreshing with hydrogen peroxide as a simple test strip shows.

The safety issues for typical pool chemicals begin immediately when added to your pool or spa. You are putting poisons and very harmful chemicals in the water. They will interact with other chemicals and organic substances to make more toxins. Each time you add pool chemicals, the concentration of toxins in the water and surrounding air equally increases. Those toxins and poisons damage your cellular body and vital organs. The air around your pool or spa, and therefore around your home, also contains these toxins and poisons that you breathe every day and every night. Day after month after year.

TO ENJOY YOUR POOL AND SPA - GET RID OF THE CHEMICALS

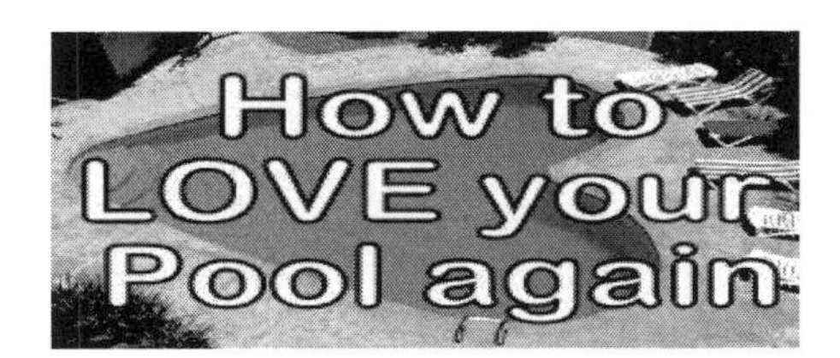

For the majority of people the health damage of chlorine and bromine is gradual but extensive throughout the whole body. Many people have strong allergic reactions to some of the chemicals in pool and spa chemicals and by the other lethal chemicals created by the reactions of those chemicals. Although not conscious of why, some people will come to so deeply dislike their spa they will leave them permanently drained or even throw them away. Others will fill-in their pool or sell their house to buy one without a pool never using it.

You cannot become allergic to hydrogen peroxide because it is only water and oxygen. A true safety distinction is that 35% food grade hydrogen peroxide becomes beneficial once added to a pool or spa. Most pool and spa chemicals start devastating your health promptly after put into your pool/spa water and make chemical laced air vapor.

HYDROGEN PEROXIDE FOR PURIFICATION OF WATER IS NOT A RARE METHOD FOR WATER PURIFICATION

Chlorine and bromine are sold as pool, spa and hot tub chemicals to people who know little to nothing about water purification. Hydrogen peroxide is used by the true professionals.

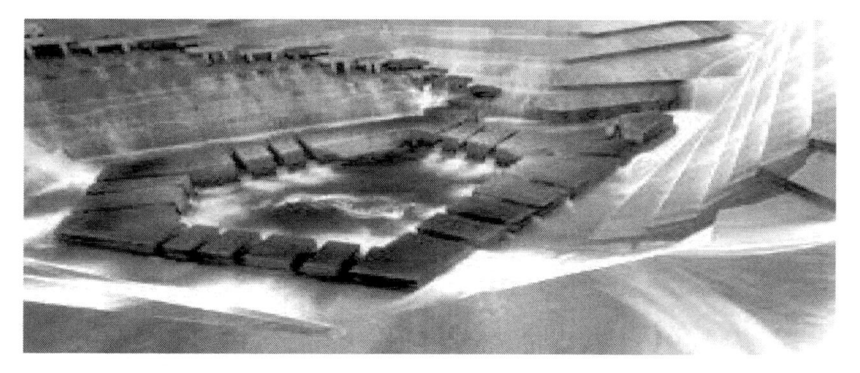

The Sensational Fort Worth Sunken Water Gardens

The Fort Worth, Texas Water Gardens cover huge. It is deeply sunken, heavily covered with old trees, and has hundreds of yards of flowing water and water curtains, ponds and fountains, which produces water vapor. They do not use chlorine or bromine. They use hydrogen peroxide. Because the area is deeply sunken there is little wind. The fumes of chlorine or bromine building in the air would be unbearable. Those chlorine based chemicals fumes would also kill the trees.

By using hydrogen peroxide there is no chemical smell. The hydrogen peroxide does not harm the vegetation. Using food grade hydrogen peroxide is such a perfect system the only clue the water is treated at all is a sticker on the door to the pump room.

When a large local urban water supply (drinking water) reached high levels of toxins and cancer-causing agents, the crisis called in the experts. To try to determine the cause, they had to test incoming water without chlorine or bromine to eliminate all the poisons and cancer causing chemicals they create when they interact with organic material. To do so, they used hydrogen peroxide to kill the organics – thus leaving only the chemicals in the water – not the organic substances. To no surprise, it was learned that it was the chlorine interacting with higher than average organic material that was causing the poisoning of the water by forming other deadly chemicals as chlorine does.

The largest chain of commercial aquariums in the U.S.A. uses 35% food grade hydrogen peroxide to treat the water in their huge aquariums – without removing the sea life and fish. While this requires expertise, treating an aquarium with the sea life still in it with chlorine or bromine would result in killing everything in the aquarium.

"A sucker is born every minute." P. T. Barnum

Chlorine and bromine are sold to home pool, spa and hot tub owners on the P.T. Barnum principle: 'A sucker born every minute". They even convince customers that somehow doing so enters the person into an exact science of water treatment - requiring endlessly testing the water's PH factors, adding chemicals, offset chemicals, balancing chemicals, anti-foaming chemicals and so forth. It is a sucker's play to do so.

More than eliminating organic growth in your pool, you want to avoid poisonous and toxic chemicals in the water. That seems obvious. I have no concerns swimming in a typical river or lake in terms of organic life in it. My only concern would be if it has dangerous chemicals. Given the choice between swimming in a river or swimming in toxic-chemical laced water, which would you choose?

Putting poisons and toxic chemicals in your pool, spa or hot tub is not what a rational person knowingly does.

If your pool or spa is terribly fouled with green growth

Some pools and spas are neglected for months and even years, resulting in terrible levels of growth fouling. This forms a thick crust, like a contaminated ship bottom. A high concentration of hydrogen peroxide will kill the growth and even will remove surface layers of it, but will not remove dense dead growth on the pool surfaces. This would allow renewed usage of the pool without further growth. There would still be the unsightly appearance but can easily be vacuumed by the pool system.

There are rare instances where an algae buildup is desirable. In those instances of decorative ponds or "pond pools" in which the pool is desired to look like a natural pond is - but also with clear and clean water. This is only possible with hydrogen peroxide, not with chlorine.

POOL SIDE PLANT LIFE

With a chlorinated pool it can be a struggle to keep plant life around a pool due to the chlorine. Pool chemical fumes kill plants. The level of dilution hydrogen peroxide for pool water is beneficial to plants. Gardeners and farmers use hydrogen peroxide for soil treatment and even plant water. The benefit is so great that if you do drain a hydrogen peroxide treated pool or spa, you may do so onto grass. Properly diluted hydrogen peroxide it is beneficial to plants.

There is no pool chemical that is beneficial to your plants. To the exact opposite, if correctly diluted 35% food grade hydrogen peroxide will help plants to thrive.

USE HYDROGEN PEROXIDE FOR YOUR POOL OR SPA

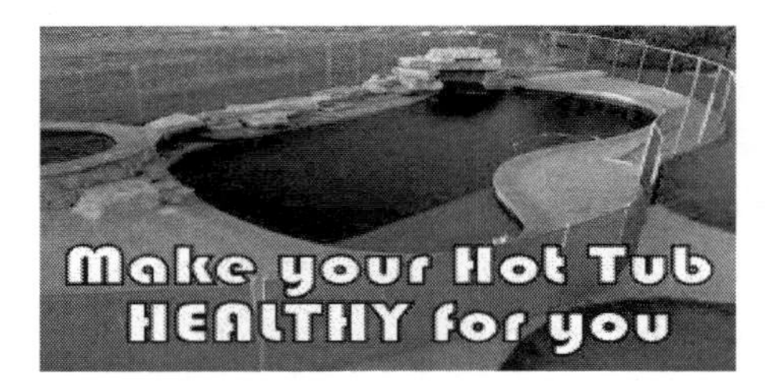

For a spa, I recommend that you first drain it to get rid of all chemicals. However, 35% food grade hydrogen peroxide will not adversely interact with current pool chemicals and some will transition to 35% food grade hydrogen peroxide usage without first draining. If your pool is highly organically fouled, you may need to use a higher initial level of 35% food grade hydrogen peroxide to kill the organics, drain this, and then go to the same maintenance levels as for a pool.

To transition to hydrogen peroxide pool care it is not necessary to drain the pool if you prefer. Or you may do so first if you want the harmful chemicals immediately eliminated. In some regions of the country water is very costly. Hydrogen peroxide does not reaction or interaction with pool chemicals. The frequency by which you add 35% food grade hydrogen peroxide will vary by the amount of organic material that comes into the water (leaves, dust, and dirt), and by what minerals are in your water; which you used a simple test strip to measure.

35% food grade hydrogen peroxide is stand-alone for pool purification, water sterilization and maintenance. You will not need any other chemicals or any other water-fixers or make any PH adjustments with hydrogen peroxide for pool and spa treatment. Unlike typical pool chemicals, there is no other chemical or substance you need to add to your poospa or hot tub **if** you use hydrogen peroxide. Eliminating toxic chemicals from damaging your cellular body is a key component in true and natural wellness.

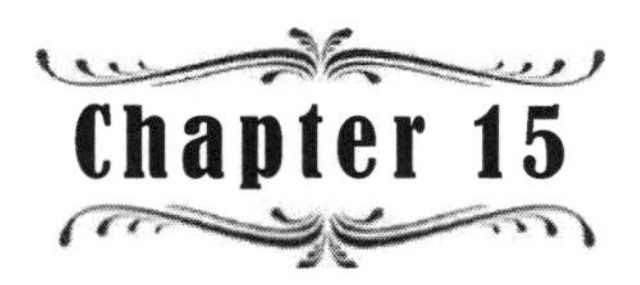

Chapter 15

Removing Chemicals From Your Home: Aromatics

> "Medicine is a collection of uncertain prescriptions, the results of which taken collectively, are more fatal than useful to mankind. Water, air and cleanliness are the chief articles in my pharmacopeia. Napoleon Bonaparte

The chemical industry and retail sales industry incessantly pushes people to buy chemicals and to use them in every way and everywhere possible. They run advertisements on television showing happy people using chemicals and even claim they improve your health.

For example, "Febreze" ™ is being put into everything claiming it eliminates odors. So are other complex manufactured chemical mixtures. They urge you to spray those chemicals in the air, on your clothes, in your car, spread it on your floor and put it in your laundry. We are bombarded with advertisements urging having chemicals constantly put into the air we breathe. Do you even know what chemicals are in them or ever bother read the label for the contents?

Many companies sell products they want you to put in your wall plug to continually put scents and chemicals into the air. Even have machines that will spray scents (meaning chemicals) at you as you walk by it. They try to sell you products to hang in your car to put in front of your vehicle's air conditioning and heater vents to put chemicals into your vehicle's interior air. There are dozens of companies that sell cans of scented chemicals they urge you to spray around your house claiming the chemicals will make your house smell cleans. Some chemicals used are so destructive they have been used for chemical weapons is more concentrated form. Others use highly toxic chemicals that essentially are pesticides.

The neurotoxins in those not only attack insects, they attack your cells through your skin and lungs. Many of these sprays also contain various oils, which build up on everything. Their motive for urging you to buy these chemical products to put into your breathing air is profit.

The human immune system is highly sensitive to odors and chemicals. Over time, most people develop increasing chemical sensitivity which increasingly triggers allergic reactions that disrupt and affect every organ in your body. Chemical and artificial odors falsely trigger defense mechanisms that can cause your body to severely react internally, externally or both. Just because there is no outward reaction you can sense, that does not mean damage is not being done internally.

Allergies cause an exaggerated response of the immune system. The immune system is an intricate system that defends the body against foreign invaders, such as bacteria and viruses, while also surveying for conditions such as cancer and autoimmunity failures to solve and eliminate the sources. Allergens are substances that are foreign to the body and can cause an allergic reaction. Most manufactured chemicals are an allergen.

An allergy refers to an exaggerated reaction by our immune system in response to exposure to certain foreign substances. It is exaggerated because these foreign substances are usually seen by the body as harmless. In allergic individuals, the body recognizes the foreign substance and the immune system generates a response which can be very adverse.

Allergy-producing substances are called "allergens." Examples of allergens include pollens, dust mites, molds, animal proteins, foods, chemicals and medications. To understand the language of allergy, it is important to remember that allergens are substances that are foreign to the body and can cause an allergic reaction. When an allergic individual comes in contact with an allergen, the immune system mounts a response through the IgE antibody. Therefore, people who are prone to allergies are said to be allergic or "atopic."

Austrian pediatrician Clemens Pirquet (1874-1929) first used the term allergy. He referred to harms to immunity by allergens and to the harmful hypersensitivity as an "allergy." The word allergy is derived from the Greek words "allos," meaning different or changed and "ergos," meaning work or action. Generally speaking, allergy therefore refers to an "altered reaction." The word allergy was first used in 1905 to describe the adverse reactions of children who were given repeated shots of horse serum to fight infection. The following year, the term allergy was proposed to explain this unexpected "changed reactivity."

Approximately 10% to 30% of individuals in the industrialized world are affected by allergic conditions.

Allergic rhinitis (nasal allergies) affects roughly 20% of Americans. Between prescription costs, physician visits, and missed days of work/school, the economic burden of allergic disease exceeds $3 billion annually. Asthma affects roughly 8% to 10% of Americans. The estimated health costs for asthma exceed approximately $20 billion annually.

The prevalence of allergic conditions has increased significantly over the last two decades and continues to rise. This is due to the increasing levels of chemicals in our air, water, and food. The parts of the body that are prone to allergic symptoms include the eyes, nose, lungs, skin, and gastrointestinal tract. Although the various allergic diseases may appear different, they all result from an exaggerated immune response to foreign substances in sensitive individuals. Over time, the human body tends become increasingly sensitive to chemicals, odors, and other substances the body senses are unnatural or dangerous.

Avoid so-called air fresheners and sprays. Do not accept the advertising and marketing hype. Spraying chemicals into the air does not make your air cleaner or safer. You should eliminate chemicals in your air rather than buying products to add chemicals to your air.

If you budget allows, purchase a HEPA rated air filter system, which are inexpensive at hardware stores. Buy one with filters that do not have scents they put out. Read the box carefully to avoid those.

The best air in your home is pure fresh air with the highest oxygen level and as few contaminants and toxins as you can prevent.

Chapter 16

Decline in Food Quality

"Health is the most valuable Possession"
Hippocrates - The Father of Medicine

In the 1950s, agricultural agencies warned that agricultural land was depleted of minerals. Plants cannot produce minerals. Plants obtain minerals by pulling minerals out of the soil. In a natural cycle, these return to the ground with each generation of plants as the old generation would fall and decompose the minerals back into the soil. Due to decades of agricultural use in which the decayed plants do not return to the soil, the soil becomes depleted of minerals in our food supply.

Once the minerals in the soil are depleted the minerals are gone. While the plants will still grow in short life spans, they are devoid of minerals with each generation. At grocery stores you can note the lack of identifying minerals in vegetables and fruit. If you read the label or mineral content specifics even for fresh fruits, grains and vegetables you can see that there are little to no mineral value in the food we eat.

The understanding of the necessity of these vital nutrients for health, energy and even mental process dates back to ancient Rome, Greece and Egypt; when it was understood that the best grains came from river deltas. Every year the soil is replenished in annual river flow in which minerals and nutrients are washed down river to settle on the delta. Animals instinctively seek out mineral rich rocks to lick and the longest lived people in the world either eat food from areas of land revived by nature or by the sea.

Incredibly, farmers and ranchers feed their livestock better than most people eat. Decades ago they learned that adding mineral supplements to their livestock's diet increases their production, growth, and health. Many farmers and ranchers have started adding 35% food grade hydrogen peroxide in trace amounts in their livestock's water. This dramatically reduces the rate of infections and helps keep the water bacteria free. Many top horse breeders add hydrogen peroxide to their horses' water. It is wise idea to do so for your pets too.

Unfortunately, no matter how well you shop at a grocery store, you cannot buy food, even vegetables and fruits, with sufficient mineral content.

These are the minerals your cells need:

Antimony	Dysprosium	Samarium	Thorium
Barium	Erbium	Scandium	Thulium
Beryllium	Europium	Selenium	Tin
Bismuth	Gadolinium	Silicon	Titanium
Boron	Gallium	Sodium	Tungsten
Cadmium	Germanium	Strontium	Vanadium
Calcium	Praseodymium	Sulfur	Ytterbium
Carbon	Rhenium	Tantalum	Yttrium
Chromium	Rhodium	Tellurium	Zinc
Cobalt	Rubidium	Terbium	Zirconium
Copper	Ruthenium	Thallium	

When people ate natural foods from non-commercial agriculture land, water and sea, their food had those minerals. Commercial agricultural land was depleted long ago of both essential primary and trace minerals.

How obtain essential trace minerals:

- Take a liquid trace mineral supplement.
- Replace table salt with a quality natural sea salt.
- Bathe in a sea salt bath occasionally. This also is beneficial to your skin.

Assuring your cells and vital organs have sufficient minerals is so easy to do it is difficult to understand why so many people neglect this obvious necessity. Do not be one of those people.

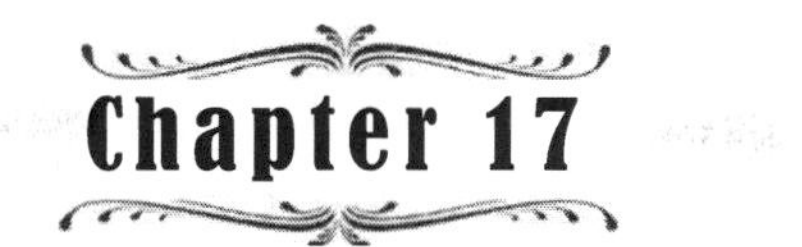

Chapter 17

Hydrogen Peroxide In Bathwater

Many benefits result from adding 35% Food Grade Hydrogen Peroxide to your bath water. It oxygenates your skin – the largest organ of the human body. It kills micro-organisms and many forms of mites on your skin and living in your skin. It helps remove dead skin and debris from your skin. Many people add hydrogen peroxide to their bath and foot bath water for health reasons. 35% food grade hydrogen peroxide oxygenates the skin and helps to clean skin (skin is porous and excretes toxic wastes). Hydrogen peroxide also eliminates fungus and other micro-organisms that live on and just below skin surface.

An example of how the skin functions is the example of how smoking damage skin. There are toxins in cigarettes and the skin tries to excrete those. The constant flow of toxins through the skin damages the skin across time. If a person is trying to quit smoking, it is advisable to frequently shower with soap to wash off the nicotine and toxins off the skin to avoid their reabsorption as the body removes such toxins through the skin. If a person is having cosmetic surgery the person is urged to stop smoking to prevent the toxins of smoking from preventing proper healing of the skin.

HOW HYDROGEN PEROXIDE WORKS AGAINST HARMFUL MICRO-ORGANIC SUBSTANCES

bath [bäth] *-noun;*
a place to wash worries away · serenity

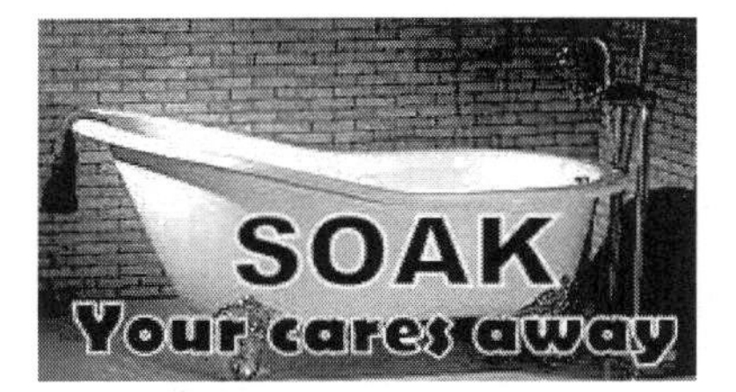

Hydrogen peroxide has been called a "kamikaze" or "depth charge" chemical against organic substances. 35% food grade hydrogen peroxide is simply water (h2o) with an extra oxygen molecule loosely attached to the h2o to make it h2o2 (hydrogen peroxide). When 35% food grade hydrogen peroxide contacts any organic molecule, the contact knocks off the extra oxygen molecule.

The result is two-fold. First, energy is released. Though certainly not noticeable as this occurs at the atomic/molecular level, the power in "decomposing" 35% food grade hydrogen peroxide is so great that hydrogen peroxide has been used to power rockets into space. 35% food grade hydrogen peroxide powered the X-15 first subsonic jet and the U.S.S.R. supersonic attack torpedoes. When the atom breaks free, the kinetic energy holding that atom is released, resulting in a flash of steam heat. The first way the hydrogen peroxide purifies is to blow up the harmful micro-organic molecule or organism.

The free oxygen atom then impacts the organic molecule, resulting in burning the molecule. Certain harmful organic substances in contact with pure oxygen "burn" (or more precisely oxidize.) The combined result is that the harmful micro-organism is blown up and "burned."

What remains of the hydrogen peroxide atom after decomposition? It is now only pure water (h2o - 2 hydrogen atoms and one oxygen atoms) and pure oxygen (0). It destroys the organic substance and then converts itself to pure water and pure oxygen in the process. That process is one of nature's miracles.

Do not shampoo with your mineral soaking bath. Briefly shower after you bath and shampoo then if you wish.

WHAT TO ADD TO BATH WATER?

In this order of priorities:

- 2 cups of 35% Food Grade Hydrogen Peroxide
- Sea salt (such as Dead Sea Salt)
- 1-2 Cups of Magnesium (such as Epson Salt)

Magnesium health supplementing is inexpensive and has remarkable health benefits. To add magnesium to your bathwater add one fourth to one half a pound of Epson salt.

If you are not already taking an oral magnesium supplement, do so. However magnesium is best absorbed through your skin the same as many other minerals. Not only is magnesium excellent for your physical and mental wellbeing, it also relaxes your muscles.

The many benefits of magnesium are discussed in a following chapter. The reason to use sea salt is also for trace mineral supplementing. The great lack in people's diets is in trace minerals. These are no longer in our food as agricultural land was stripped of minerals years ago. Plants can make vitamins, but not minerals. See chapter 17 for the benefits of magnesium.

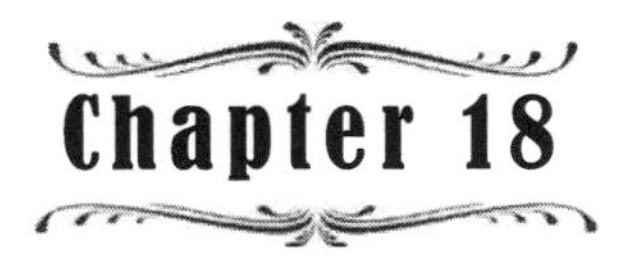

Chapter 18

The Benefits of Magnesium

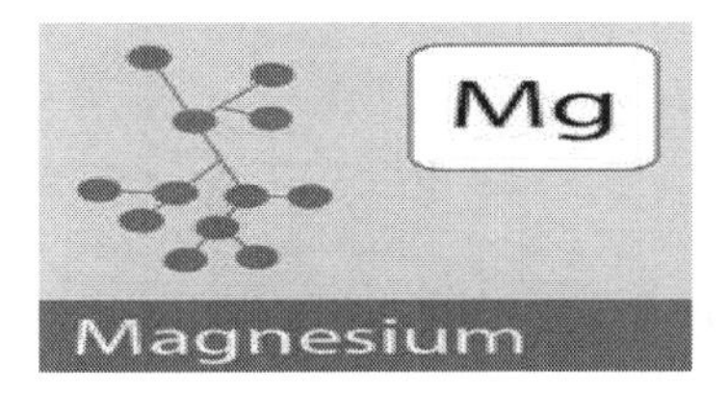

By adding 35% food grade hydrogen peroxide to your bath water – the hydrogen peroxide will cleanse your skin of harmful fungus, bacteria, micro-organisms, and will oxygenate your skin – as will magnesium. You should add magnesium as an oral supplement (tablet) for how critical and beneficial it is.

The Benefits of sufficient Magnesium, curative effects of Magnesium supplementing, and dangers of Magnesium deficiency has been established by formal medical studies across the globe. Studies and results listed in the text of this book and in the Bibliography include from the USA, France, Germany, Japan, Great Britain, South Africa, Netherlands, Denmark, Hungary and Switzerland.

This incredible list includes mainstream and alternative healthcare experts and medical researchers and facilities. What follows is long and technical.

You may wish to skip the rest of this chapter. But the material is added to as samples show you the many tremendous significant benefits of magnesium supplementing – and the very real dangers of magnesium deficiency. If you skip reading this chapter, do not skip the importance of magnesium in your health supplementation.

Magnesium and carbohydrate metabolism
THERAPIE (France), 1994, 49/1 (1-7)

The interrelationships between magnesium and carbohydrate metabolism have regained considerable interest over the last few years. Insulin secretion requires magnesium: magnesium deficiency results in impaired insulin secretion while magnesium replacement **restores insulin secretion.** Furthermore, experimental magnesium **deficiency reduces the tissues sensitivity to insulin.** Sub clinical magnesium deficiency is common in diabetesIn type 2, or non-insulin- dependent, diabetes mellitus, magnesium deficiency seems to be associated with insulin resistance. Furthermore, it may participate in the pathogenesis of **diabetes complications** and may contribute to the increased risk of sudden death associated with diabetes. Some studies suggest that magnesium deficiency may play a role in spontaneous abortion of diabetic women, in fetal malformations and in the pathogenesis of **neonatal hypocalcemia of the infants of diabetic mothers.** Administration of magnesium salts to patients with type 2 diabetes tend to **reduce insulin resistance.** Long-term studies are needed before recommending systematic magnesium supplementation to type 2 diabetic patients with subclinical magnesium deficiency.

Disorders of magnesium metabolism

Endocrinology and Metabolism Clinics of North America (USA), 1995, 24/3

Magnesium depletion is more common than previously thought. It seems to be especially prevalent in patients with **diabetes** mellitus. It is usually caused by losses from the kidney or gastrointestinal tract. A patient with magnesium depletion may present with **neuromuscular, hypokalemia, hypocalcemia, or cardiovascular complications. Physicians should maintain a high index of suspicion for magnesium depletion and should implement therapy early.**

Magnesium deficiency produces insulin resistance and increased thromboxane synthesis

HYPERTENSION (USA), 1993, 21/6 II (1024-1029)

Evidence suggests **that magnesium deficiency may play an importantvrole in cardiovascular disease.** In this study, we evaluated the effects of a magnesium infusion and dietary-induced isolated magnesium deficiency on the production of thromboxane and on angiotensin II- mediated aldosterone synthesis in normal human subjects. Because insulin resistance may be associated with altered blood pressure, we also measured insulin sensitivity using an intravenous glucose tolerance test with minimal model analysis in six subjects. The magnesium infusion **reduced urinary thromboxane**

concentration and angiotensin II-induced plasma aldosterone levels. The low magnesium diet reduced both serum magnesium and intracellular free magnesium in red blood cells as determined by nuclear magnetic resonance (186plus or minus10 (SEM) to 127plus or minus9 mM, p<0.01). Urinary thromboxane concentration measured by radioimmunoassay increased after magnesium deficiency. Similarly, angiotensin II- induced plasma aldosterone concentration increased after magnesium deficiency.

Analysis showed that all subjects studied had a **decrease in insulin sensitivity** after magnesium deficiency (3.69plus or minus0.6 to 2.75plus or minus0.5 min- 1 per microunit per milliliterx10-4, p<0.03). We conclude that dietary- induced magnesium deficiency 1) increases thromboxane urinary concentration and 2) enhances angiotensin- induced aldosterone synthesis. These effects are associated with a decrease in insulin action, suggesting that magnesium deficiency may be a common factor associated with **insulin resistance and vascular disease.**

Magnesium and glucose homeostasis
DIABETOLOGIA (Germany, Federal Republic of), 1990, 33/9 (511-514)
Magnesium is an important ion in all living cells being a cofactor of many enzymes, especially those utilizing high energy phosphate bounds. The relationship between insulin and magnesium has been recently studied. In particular it has been shown that magnesium plays the role of a second messenger for insulin action; on the other hand, insulin itself has been demonstrated to be an important regulatory factor of intracellular magnesium accumulation. Conditions associated with insulin resistance, such as hypertension or aging, are also associated with low intracellular magnesium contents. In diabetes mellitus, it is suggested that low intracellular magnesium levels result from both increased urinary losses and insulin resistance. The extent to which such low intracellular magnesium content contributes to the development of macro- and microangiopathy remains to be established. Reduced intracellular magnesium content might contribute to the impaired insulin response and action which occurs in Type 2 (non- insulin-dependent) diabetes mellitus.
Chronic magnesium supplementation can contribute to an improvement in both islet **Beta- cell response and insulin action** in non-insulin-dependent diabetes subjects.

Magnesium content of erythrocytes in patients with vasospastic angina

CARDIOVASC. DRUGS THER. (USA), 1991, 5/4 (677-680)

The possibility that a magnesium deficiency might be the underlying cause of vasospastic angina (VA) and the efficacy of Mg administration in its treatment were studied. Subjects included 15 patients with VA and 18 healthy subjects as the control group. The erythrocyte Mg content was measured by atomic absorption, and serum Mg was measured by conventional chemical assay. The efficacy of Mg administration was studied in seven patients with VA. The results were as follows: (a) The mean erythrocyte Mg content was less in the group with frequent episodes of angina (1.59 plus or minus 0.11 mg/dl) than in the group without angina (2.11 plus or minus 0.38 mg/dl, $p < 0.01$) and in the control group (2.22 plus or minus 0.29 mg/dl, $p < 0.01$). There was no significant difference between the control group and patients of each group with respect to serum Mg. (b) Coronary arterial spasm was induced by ergonovine maleate in seven patients and was completely inhibited by the administration of Mg sulfate (40-80 mEq, hourly) in six of these patients; in the remaining patient neither obvious ST change nor chest pain occurred. Thus, it was concluded that the measurement of erythrocyte Mg content is useful to determine how easily vasospasm might occur in VA and that the administration of Mg might be developed as **a new therapy for spasm** associated with low erythrocyte Mg content.

Variant angina due to deficiency of intracellular magnesium

CLIN. CARDIOL. (USA), 1990, 13/9 (663-665)

A 51-year-old man was diagnosed as having variant angina by documentation of typical ST elevation during 82ehavi attack and also by **showing coronary arterial spasm** (#2 and #12) during hyperventilation on coronary arteriography. Large quantities of calcium blocking agents and nitrates could not improve his symptoms. Lack of intracellular magnesium was suspected from a daily excretion of urine magnesium (5.3 mEq) and magnesium tolerance test (56.7%). After hourly infusion of magnesium sulfate (80 mEq), coronary spasm could not be induced by ergonovine.

Magnesium deficiency and sudden death

S. AFR. MED. J. (SOUTH AFRICA), 1983, 64/18 (697-698)

Magnesium deficiency may result from reduced dietary intake of the ion increased losses in sweat, urine or feces. Stress potentiates magnesium deficiency, and an increased incidence of sudden death associated with ischaemic heart disease is found in some areas in which soil and drinking water lack magnesium. Furthermore, it has been demonstrated experimentally **that reduction of the plasma magnesium level is associate with arterial spasm.** Careful studies are required to assess the clinical importance of magnesium and the benefits of magnesium supplementation in man.

Magnesium deficiency produces spasms of coronary arteries: Relationship to etiology of sudden death ischemic heart disease
SCIENCE (USA), 1980, 208/4440 (198-200)
Isolated coronary arteries from dogs were incubated in Krebs-Ringer bicarbonate solution and exposed to normal, high, and low concentrations of magnesium in the medium. Sudden withdrawal of magnesium from the medium increased whereas **high concentrations of magnesium decreased the basal tension of the arteries.** The absence of magnesium in the medium significantly potentiated the contractile responses of both small and large coronary arteries to norepinephrine, acetylcholine, serotonin, angiotensin, and potassium. These data support that magnesium deficiency, associated with sudden death ischemic heart disease, produces coronary arterial spasm.

Magnesium and potassium in diabetes and carbohydrate metabolism. Review of the present status and recent results.

Magnesium 1984. 3(4-6). P 315-23
Diabetes mellitus is the most common pathological state in which secondary magnesium deficiency occurs. Magnesium metabolism abnormalities vary according to the multiple clinical forms of diabetes: plasma magnesium is more often decreased than red blood cell magnesium. Plasma Mg levels are correlated mainly with the severity of the diabetic state, glucose disposal and endogenous insulin secretion. Various mechanisms are involved in the induction of Mg depletion in diabetes mellitus, i.e. insulin and epinephrine secretion, modifications of the vitamin D metabolism, decrease of blood P, vitamin B6 and taurine levels, increase of vitamin B5, C and glutathione turnover, treatment with high levels of insulin and biguanides. K depletion in diabetes mellitus is well known.

Some of its mechanisms are concomitant to those of Mg depletion. But their hierarchic importance is not the same: i.e., insulin hyposecretion is more important versus K+ than versus Mg2+. Insulin increases the cellular inflow of K+ more than that of Mg2+ because there is more free K+ (87%) than Mg2+ (30%) in the cell. The consequences of the double Mg-K depletion are either antagonistic: i.e. versus insulin secretion (increased by K+, decreased by Mg2+) or agonistic i.e. on the membrane: (i.e. Na+K+ATPase), tolerance of glucose oral load, renal disturbances. The real importance of these disorders in the diabetic condition is still poorly understood. Retinopathy and microangiopathy are correlated with the drop of plasma and red blood cell Mg. K deficiency increases the noxious cardiorenal effects of Mg deficiency. The treatment should primarily insure diabetic control.

Hypocalcemia associated with estrogen therapy for metastatic adenocarcinoma of the prostate

J. UROL. (USA), 1988, 140/5 PART I (1025-1027)

We report 2 cases of true hypocalcemia (not caused by decreased binding protein) associated with metastatic prostate cancer and review previously reported cases. Hypocalcemia is a common but frequently unrecognized complication of **prostatic cancer**. Estrogen therapy often is associated with the hypocalcemia, which may be asymptomatic. The hypocalcemia is always associated with osteoblastic metastases and usually it is associated with increased serum alkaline phosphatase activity, acid phosphatase activity and serum parathyroid hormone concentration. Serum concentrations of magnesium, phosphorus and vitamin D frequently are decreased. Patients are in a positive calcium balance. The osteoblastic metastases seem to act as a calcium sink, creating a 'hungry tumor phenomenon'. The role of estrogens may be to stop the resorption of normal bone resulting in lower serum calcium concentrations.

[Overview–suppression effect of essential trace elements on arteriosclerotic development and its mechanism]

Arteriosclerosis

Saito N/Nippon Rinsho (JAPAN) Jan 1996, 54 (1) p59-66

It is known that the peroxidation of LDL is a trigger for developing **arteriosclerosis**. The oxidized LDL is produced by either oxidative stress or a few oxidants. Selenium decreased in serum and some organs of stroke-prone spontaneously hypertensive rats (SHRSP), which is a cofactor of glutamine peroxidase. Serum magnesium decreased in patients with diabetes mellitus, with ischemic heart disease, with essential hypertension and with cerebral vascular lesions. Calcium to in SHRSP. (21 Refs.)

Magnesium hormonal regulation and metabolic interrelations
PRESSE MED. (France), 1988, 17/12 (584-587)
Magnesium ion is of great importance in physiology by its intervention in 300 enzymatic systems, its role in membrane structure and its function in neuromuscular excitability. The skeleton is the first pool of magnesium in the body. Intestinal absorption, renal metabolism, bone accretion and resorption of magnesium are very similar to those of calcium. Magnesium metabolism is accurately controlled, in particular by parathyroid hormone, 25 – dihydroxy vitamin D3, calcitonin, catecholamine and estrogens. The main regulation mechanisms of magnesium metabolism are located in the **kidney** which is the principal excretory organ.

Magnesium deficiency: Possible role in osteoporosis associated with gluten-sensitive enteropathy

Osteoporosis International (United Kingdom), 1996, 6/6 (453-461)
Osteoporosis and magnesium (Mg) deficiency often occur in malabsorption syndromes such as gluten-sensitive enteropathy (GSE). Mg deficiency is known to **impair parathyroid hormone** (PTH) **secretion and action in humans and will result in osteopenia and increased skeletal fragility** in animal models. We hypothesize that Mg depletion may contribute to the osteoporosis associated with malabsorption. It was our objective to determine Mg status and bone mass in GSE patients who were clinically asymptomatic and on a stable gluten-free diet, as well as their response to Mg therapy. Twenty-three patients with biopsy-proven GSE on a gluten-free diet were assessed for Mg deficiency by determination of the serum Mg, red blood cell (RBC) and lymphocyte free Mg^{2+}, and total lymphocyte Mg. Fourteen subjects completed a 3-month treatment period in which they were given 504-576 mg $MgCl_2$ or Mg lactate daily. Serum PTH, 25- hydroxyvitamin D, 1,25-dihydroxyvitamin D and osteocalcin were measured at baseline and monthly thereafter. Eight patients who had documented Mg depletion (RBC $Mg^{2+} < 150$ microM) underwent bone density measurements of the lumbar spine and proximal femur, and 5 of these patients were followed for 2 years on Mg therapy. The mean serum Mg, calcium, phosphorus and alkaline phosphatase concentrations were in the normal range.

Most serum calcium values fell below mean normal and the baseline serum PTH was high normal or slightly elevated in 7 of the 14 subjects who completed the 3-month treatment period. No correlation with the serum calcium was noted, however. Mean serum 25-hydroxyvitamin D, 1,25-dihydroxy vitamin D and osteocalcin concentrations were also normal. Despite only 1 patient having hypomagnesemia, the RBC Mg2+ (153 + or – 6.2 microM; mean plus or minus SEM) and lymphocyte Mg2+ (182 plus or minus 5.5 microM) were significantly lower than normal (202 + or – 6.0 microM, $P < 0.001$, and 198 + or – 6.8 microM, $p < 0.05$, respectively).

Bone densitometry revealed that 4 of 8 patients had **osteoporosis** of the lumbar spine and 5 of 8 had osteoporosis of the proximal femur (T-scores less than or equal to -2.5). Mg therapy resulted in a significant rise in the mean serum PTH concentration from 44.6 + or – 3.6 pg/ml to 55.9 plus or minus 5.6 pg/ml ($p < 0.05$). In the 5 patients given Mg supplements for 2 years, a significant increase in bone mineral density was observed in the femoral neck and total proximal femur. This **increase in bone mineral density** correlated positively with a rise in RBC Mg2+. This study demonstrates that GSE patients have reduction in intracellular free Mg2+, despite being clinically asymptomatic on a gluten-free diet. Bone mass also appears to be reduced. Mg therapy resulted in a rise in PTH, suggesting that the intracellular Mg deficit was impairing PTH secretion in these patients. **The increase in bone density in response to Mg therapy suggests that Mg depletion may be one factor contributing to osteoporosis**.

Energy and nutrient intake in patients with CF
Monatsschrift fur Kinderheilkunde (Germany),1996,144/4 (396-402)

Background: Nutritional assessment and management remain important issues in the treatment of CF patients despite newer developments as lung transplantation, inhalation with Dnase and gene therapy. Methods: The nutritional status of 26 patients (mean age 15,8 years; 16 male; 46% homozygous, 38% heterozygous for DeltaF 508, remaining unknown; 3 pancreas sufficient, Shwachman score intermediate to excellent) of our CF clinic was analyzed using a three days protocol, the precise weighing method and comparison of data with the official dietary recommendations.

The average energy intake was below 130% officially recommended and the fat intake was below the aimed 40% of total energy intake. The regression analysis revealed positive correlations between energy intake and SDS(Height) and Shwachman score and SDS(Weight) respectively. Food contained an insufficient amount of unsaturated fatty acids. Water soluble vitamins were supplemented adequately besides folic acid, but intake of fat soluble vitamins E and A often was insufficient despite extra vitamin capsules. Every second patient did not take enough minerals as calcium magnesium or iron.

Conclusions: **This analysis underlines how important the regular assessment of the nutritional status can be for the individual nutrit ional management of CF patients even if clinical symptoms of deficiencies could not be detected.** An increase of fat intake as a main source of energy, essential fatty acids and soluble vitamins has to be encouraged as well as the increased use of milk and milk products for the prevention of osteoporosis. Iron and folic acid are further critical nutrients.

Kidney stone clinic: Ten years of experience
Nederlands Tijschrift voor de Klinische Chemie (Netherlands), 1996, 21/1 (8-10)

Experiences are described at a **kidney stone** clinic which was established as part of the Department of Clinical Biochemistry ten years ago. During this period, the investigational protocol has changed from an in-patient to an out-patient scheme. The most important metabolic abnormalities among calcium oxalate **kidney stone** formers were hypercalciuria, hypernatriuria, hyperuricosuria, increased blood urate, decreased blood phosphate and hyperphosphaturia with decreased renal phosphate threshold. These abnormalities were found in the majority of patients. Oxalate output was, however, increased in less than 50 percent of the patients. The effectivity of thiazides, allopurinol, magnesium and phosphate supplementation was tested, and it was concluded that (a) the effect of thiazides was significant, but calciuria normalized only in a few cases, (b) the withdrawal of allopurinol led to a significant increase of urate parameters only in patients without a low-purine diet, (c) a sufficient dose of magnesium and phosphate is necessary to achieve a therapeutie effect. **Preliminar y data indicate that some patients with hypercalciuria and kidney stones are at risk of decreased bone mass,** and the role of bone markers monitoring is mentioned.

Plasma copper, zinc and magnesium levels in patients with premenstrual tension syndrome.

ACTA OBSTET. GYNECOL. SCAND. (Denmark), 1994, 73/6 (452-455)

We measured plasma Cu, Zn and Mg levels in 40 women suffering from **premenstrual tension syndrome (PMTS)** and in 20 control subjects by atomic absorption spectrophotometer. Mean plasma Cu, Zn and Mg levels, the Zn/Cu ratio were 80.2 plus or minus 6.00 microg/dl, 112.6 plus or minus 8.35 microg/dl, 0.70 plus or minus 0.18 mmol/l, and 1.40 plus or minus 0.10 in the PMTS group; and 77.0 plus or minus 4.50 microg/dl, 117.4 plus or minus 9.50 microg/dl, 0.87 plus or minus 0.10 mmol/l, and 1.51 plus or minus 0.05 in the control group respectively. The mean Mg level and the Zn/Cu ratio were significantly lower in PMTS patients than in the control group. Plasma Mg and Zn levels were diminished significantly during the luteal phase compared to the follicular phase in PMTS group. Mg deficiency may play a role in the etiology of PMTS.

Oral magnesium successfully relieves premenstrual mood changes OBSTET. GYNECOL. (USA), 1991, 78/2 (177-181)

Reduced magnesium (Mg) levels have been reported in women affected by premenstrual syndrome (PMS). To evaluate the effects of an oral Mg preparation on premenstrual symptoms, we studied, by a double-blind, randomized design, 32 women (24-39 years old) with PMS confirmed by the Moos Menstrual Distress Questionnaire. In the next two cycles, both groups received Mg. Magnesium pyrro lidone carboxylic acid (360 mg Mg) or placebo was administered three times a day, from the 15th day of the menstrual cycle to the onset of menstrual flow. Blood samples for Mg measurement were drawn premenstrually, during the baseline period, and in the second and fourth months of treatment. The Menstrual Distress Questionnaire score of the cluster 'pain' was significantly reduced during the second month in both groups, whereas Mgc treatments significantly affected both the total Menstrual Distress Questionnaire score and the cluster 'negative affect'. In the second month, the women assigned to treatment showed a significant increase in Mg in lymphocytes and polymer-phonuclear cells, whereas no changes were observed in plasma and erythrocytes. These data indicate that Mg (magnesium) supplementation could represent **an effective treatment of premenstrual symptoms** related to mood changes.

Magnesium and the premenstrual syndrome

ANN. CLIN. BIOCHEM. (UK), 1986, 23/6 (667-670)

Plasma and erythrocyte magnesium were measured in 105 patients with **premenstrual syndro me (PMS)** using a simple atomic absorption spectroscopy method. The erythrocyte magnesium concentration for the patients with PMS was significantly lower than that of a normal population. The plasma magnesium did not show this difference. The significant of this apparent cellular deficiency of magnesium is discussed.

Magnesium concentration in brains from multiple sclerosis patients

ACTA NEUROL. SCAND. (Denmark), 1990, 81/3 (197-200)

Magnesium (Mg) concentrations were studied in the brains of 4 patients with definite **multiple sclerosis** (MS) and 5 controls. The magnesium contents were determined by inductively coupled plasma emission spectrometry in autopsy samples taken from 26 sites of central nervous system tissues, and visceral organs such as liver, spleen, kidney, heart and lung. The average Mg content in the CNS tissues, as well as visceral organs except for spleen, of MS patients showed a significantly lower value than that seen in control cases. The most marked reduction of Mg content was observed in CNS white matter including demyelinated plaques of MS samples. Whether or not these significantly lower Mg contents found in CNS and visceral organs of MS patients may play an essential role in the demyelinating process remain unclear, requiring further studies on MS pathogenesis from the point of metal metabolism.

Zinc, copper and magnesium concentration in serum and CSF of patients with **neurological disorders**

ACTA NEUROL. SCAND. (Denmark), 1989, 79/5 (373-378)

Zinc (Zn), copper (Cu) and magnesium (Mg) concentrations in cerebrospinal fluid (CSF) and serum were determined with atomic absorption spectrophotometry in 74 patients suffering from various neurological diseases, and in 28 healthy controls. Increased CSF zinc levels were found in the group of peripheral **nervous system diseases** ($P < 0.01$) and in the cases of different neurological syndromes with increased CSF protein concentration ($P < 0.001$). Increased CSF and serum copper levels were found in the cases with increased CSF protein levels ($P < 0.05$). It is probable that damaged blood-brain-barrier

(BBB) permits the passage of the trace elements Zn, Cu and of Mg into the subarachnoid space. Decreased serum Cu levels ($P < 0.01$) were found in the group of multiple sclerosis (MS). The findings are correlated to those of previous communications.

The susceptibility of the centrocecal scotoma to electrolytes, especially in **multiple sclerosis**
IDEGGYOG.SZLE (HUNGARY), 1973, 26/7 (307-312)
A study of the action of magnesium on the centrocecal scotoma in multiple sclerosis revealed that the scotomas were transiently reduced by magnesium infusions or that calcium ionization was modified by alkalinization or Na EDTA.

Experimental and clinical studies on dysregulation of magnesium metabolism and the aetiopathogenesis of **multiple sclerosis.**
Magnes Res (ENGLAND) Dec 1992, 5 (4) p295-302
The proposed aetiologies of multiple sclerosis (MS) have included immunological mechanisms, genetic factors, virus infection and direct or indirect action of minerals and/or metals. The processes of these aetiologies have implicated magnesium. Magnesium and zinc have been shown to be decreased in central nervous system (CNS) tissues of MS patients, especially tissues such as white matter where pathological changes have been observed. The calcium content of white matter has also been found to be decreased in MS patients. The interactions of minerals and/or metals such as calcium, magnesium, aluminium and zinc have also been evaluated in CNS tissues of experimental animal models. These data suggest that these elements are regulated by pooling of minerals and/or metals in bones. Biological actions of magnesium may affect the maintenance and function of nerve cells as well as the proliferation and synthesis of lymphocytes.
A magnesium deficit may induce dysfunction of nerve cells or lymphocytes directly and/or indirectly, and thus magnesium depletion may be implicated in the aetiology of MS. The action of zinc helps to prevent virus infection, and zinc deficiency in CNS tissues of MS patients may also be relevant to its aetiology. **Magnesium interacts wit h other minerals and/or metals such as calcium, zinc and aluminium in biological systems, affecting the immune system** and influencing the content of these elements in CNS tissues. Because of these interactions, a magnesium deficit could also be a risk factor in the aetiology of MS. 9

Magnesium concentration in plasma and erythrocytes in MS <u>**Acta Neurologica Scandinavica**</u> **(Denmark), 1995, 92/1 (109-111)**
There are few reports of Mg in MS and none dealing with Mg content in erythrocytes. Mg concentration was determined in serum and in erythrocytes with the help of a BIOTROL Magnesium Calmagite colorimetric method (average sensitivity: 0.194 A per mmol/I) and a Hitachi auto analyzer in 24 MS patients (7 men and 17 women, age 29-60; 37 years on average with the duration of the disease: 3-19; 11 years on average, at clinical disability stages according to the Kurtzke scale: 1-7; 3.2 on average, in remission stage. A statistically significant decrease of Mg concentration in erythrocytes and no changes in plasma of MS patients were found. The results obtained suggest the presence of changes in membrane of erythrocytes which could be **connected with their shorter life** and with affection of their function.

Comparative findings on serum Img2+ of normal and diseased human subjects with the NOVA and KONE ISE's for Mg2+ <u>**SCAND. J. CLIN. LAB. INVEST. SUPPL.**</u> **(United Kingdom), 1994, 54/217**
It is clear now that although different ionophores for ionized Mg (Img2+) have been designed by several groups, each of these has a distinctly different K(MgCa). In view of this, it is important to determine whether each of these ion selective electrodes (ISE's) yield identical results for Img2+ in sera from healthy and diseased humans. Using such an approach, we determined, in a blinded-and random manner, Img2+ with both the NOVA and KONE ISE's for Img2+ in two independent laboratories. No significant differences were found either for sera from healthy human volunteers or diseased patients. We did, however, note several interesting findings: 1. Randomly, selected hospitalized patients exhibit a much higher incidence of abnormalities for Img2+ (57-71%) than that noted previously for total Mg (TMg) measurements; and 2 exhibit extracellular deficits in ionized free Mg.. **Coronary heart disease, rectal cancer and multiple sclerosis patients.**

Migraine–diagnosis, differential diagnosis and therapy
<u>**Ther Umsch**</u> **(SWITZERLAND) Feb 1997, 54 (2) p64-70**
Migraine is caused by intermittent brain dysfunction. Attacks result in severe unilateral headache with nausea, vomiting, photophobia, phonophobia and general weakness.

The prevalence of **migraine** is 12 to 20% in women and 8 to 12% in man. Treatment of an acute attack is done by antiemetics in combination with analgesics. **Severe migraine attacks** are treated with ergotamine or sumatriptan. Parenteral treatment is performed most efficiently and safely with i.v. ASA. Frequent and severe attacks require prophylaxis. Drugs of first choice are metoprolol, propranolol, flunarizine and cyclandelate. Substances of second choice are valproic acid, DHE, pizotifen, methysergide and magnesium. Homeopathic remedies are not superior to placebo. Nonpharmacological treatment consists of sport therapy and muscle relaxation techniques.

Prophylaxis of migraine with oral magnesium: results from a prospective, multi-center, placebo-controlled and double-blind randomized study.

Cephalalgia (NORWAY) Jun 1996, 16 (4) p257-63

In order to evaluate the prophylactic effect of oral magnesium, 81 patients aged 18-65 years with migraine according to the International Headache Society (IHS) criteria (mean attack frequency 3.6 per month) were examined. After a prospective baseline period of 4 weeks they received oral 600 mg (24 mmol) magnesium (trimagnesium dicitrate) daily for 12 weeks or placebo. In weeks 9-12 the attack frequency was reduced by 41.6% in the magnesium group and by 15.8% in the placebo group compared to the baseline ($p < 0.05$). The number of days with migraine and the drug consumption for symptomatic treatment per patient also decreased significantly in the magnesium group. Duration and intensity of the attacks and the drug consumption per attack also tended to decrease compared to placebo but failed to be significant. Adverse events were diarrhea (18.6%) and gastric irritation (4.7%). **High-dose oral magnesium appears to be effective in migraine prophylaxis.**

Electromyographical ischemic test and intracellular and extracellular magnesium concentration in migraine and tension-type headache patients.

Headache (UNITED STATES) Jun 1996, 36 (6) p357-61

Headache has often been described in the hyperexcitability syndrome which recognizes an alteration of calcium and magnesium status in its etiopathogenesis. Moreover, in **migraine patients** magnesium has been shown to play an important role as a regulator of neuronal excitability and, therefore hypothetically, of headache. The present research involves a neurophysiological evaluation and magnesium status assessment of a group of headache patients. Nineteen patients (15 women and 4 men) with episodic tension-type headache and 30 patients (27 women and 3 men) with migraine without aura were examined. An ischemic test was carried out on the right arm with electromyographic (EMG) recording of motor unit potential activity during the interictal period. The determination of extracellular (serum and saliva) and intracellular (red and mononuclear blood cells) magnesium was also performed. **The EMG test was positive** in 25 of 30 migraine patients and in 2 of 19 tension-type headache patients.

Between the two patient groups, there were no significant variations in the concentration of extracellular and white blood cell magnesium, while the red blood cell concentration of this mineral in the group of migraineurs was significantly reduced with respect to that in the group of tension-type headache patients ($P < 0.05$). The positive EMG test was significantly associated with a low concentration of red blood cell magnesium ($P < 0.0001$). These results confirm previous findings by demonstrating different etiopathogenic mechanisms as the basis of migraine and tension-type headache. Migraine seems to be related to an altered magnesium status, which manifests itself by a neuromuscular hyperexcitability and a reduced concentration in red blood cells.

Magnesium supplementation and osteoporosis
Nutrition Reviews (USA), 1995, 53/3 (71-74)
Among other things, magnesium regulates active calcium transport. As a result, there has been a growing interest in the role of magnesium (Mg) in **bone metabolism.** A group of menopausal women were given magnesium hydroxide to assess the effects of magnesium on bone density. At the end of the 2-year study, magnesium therapy appears to have prevented fractures and resulted in a significant increase in bone density.

Calcium, phosphorus and magnesium intakes correlate with bone mineral content in postmenopausal women GYNECOL. ENDOCRINOL. (United Kingdom), 1994, 8/1 (55-58)

Qualitative and quantitative differences in the dietary habits of postmenopausal women were studied to assess their influence on bone health and osteoporosis. A total of 194 **postmenopausal women** were studied with forearm DEXA densitometry. 70 were osteoporotic and served as controls. Women had been menopausal for had never been treated with hormone replacement or drug therapy. A 3- day dietary recall was completed on Sunday, Monday and Tuesday after the examination: the results were processed by computer and daily calcium, phosphorus and magnesium intakes were related to bone mineral content (BMC). Data were compared with Student's t-test and significance was assessed at $p < 0.05$. Regression analysis was performed to correlate BMC and intake levels.

The dietary intake of calcium phosphorus and magnesium was significantly reduced in osteoporotic women and correlated with BMC. Calcium and magnesium intakes were lower than the recommended daily allowance even in normal women. The results suggest that nutritional factors are relevant to bone health in post menopausal women, and dietary supplementation may be indicated for the prophylaxis of osteoporosis. Adequate nutritional recommendations and supplements should be given before the menopause, and dietary evaluation should be mandatory in treating postmenopausal osteoporosis.

Magnesium in the physiopathology and treatment of renal calcium stones

PRESSE MED. (FRANCE), 1987, 16/1 (25-27)

The inhibitory effect of magnesium on the first stages of **renal calcium stone formation** is modest in vitro and more pronounced in experimental in vivo studies. Magnesium deficiency has not yet been convincingly demonstrated in man. However, urinary magnesium concentrations are abnormally low in relation to urinary calcium concentrations in more than 25% of patients with kidney stones. A supplementary magnesium intake corrects this abnormality and prevents the recurrence of stones. Magnesium seems to be as effective against stone formation as diuretics. The modalities of magnesium therapy still have to be determined and its results confirmed. **Magnesium, possibly added to drinking water, may well play a role in the primary prevention of renal calcium stones**.

Urinary factors of kidney stone formation in patients with Crohn's disease KLIN. WOCHENSCHR. (Germany, Federal Republic of), 1988, 66/3v(87-91)

An increased frequency of **kidney stone** formation is reported in patients with inflammatory bowel disease. In order to investigate its pathogenesis, the concentrations of factors known to enhance calcium oxalate stone formation (oxalate, calcium, uric acid) as well as of inhibitory factors for nephrolithiasis (magnesium, citrate) were determined in the urine of 86 patients with **Crohn's disease** and compared with those of 53 metabolically healthy controls.

Six patients with **Crohn's disease** already had experienced calciu m oxalate nephro lithiasis. Patients with **Crohn's disease** had significant ly higher urinary oxalate and lower magnesium and citrate concentrations. Among all patients magnesium and citrate were significantly lower in those with a positive history of kidney stones. Our results demonstrate that the increased propensity for **renal stone formation** in patients with Crohn's disease is a result not only of increased urinary oxalate, but also of decreased urinary magnesium and citrate concentrations.

Renal stone formation in patients with inflammatory bowel disease

SCANNING MICROSC. (USA), 1993, 7/1 (371-380)

Kidney stones are more common in patients with inflammatory bowel disease (IBD) than in the general population.

The main lithogenetic risk factors were evaluated in patients affected by **Crohn's** disease and ulcerative colitis. Our results show the presence of several factors, besides hyperoxaluria, in patients with IBD although their behavior appears different in **Crohn's disease** and ulcerative colitis at pre- and post-operative stages. Before surgery in patients with Crohn's disease we found a decreased citrate ($p < 0.001$) and magnesium ($p < 0.005$) excretion together with a low urinary volume ($p < 0.001$) and pH ($p < 0.005$). After surgery patients with Crohn's disease showed a further reduction of magnesium and citrate. Patients with ulcerative colitis before surgery showed a reduced citrate excretion ($p < 0.05$) and a more acidic pH ($p < 0.05$) than healthy subjects.

Surgical treatment of proctocolectomy with ileal pouch-ana l anastomosis seems to increase the risk of stone formation; in fact, after surgery we observed a relevant decrease of urinary volume ($p < 0.001$), pH ($p < 0.0001$) and urinary excretion of citrate ($p < 0.0001$) as well as magnesium ($p < 0.005$). Patients with IBD seem to be at greater risk of stone formation than patients with idiopathic calcium lithiasis; in fact, they show a lower excretion of citrate ($p < 0.001$) and magnesium ($p < 0.001$) together with a low urinary pH ($p < 0.001$) and volume ($p < 0.001$). Urinary volume reduction is probably one of the major risk factors together with the decrease of small molecular weight inhibitors that is a constant finding in all patients with IBD.

Did the above convince you to make certain you are not deficient in Magnesium?

The studies above collectively present the great importance to have a sufficient Magnesium intake. Magnesium is a necessary mineral to process calcium, in physical and mental process, in 300 enzymatic systems, in membrane structure and in the neuromuscular system and in proper kidney functions. They clearly establish that Magnesium is a cornerstone mineral in virtually every human body function.

Magnesium is both inexpensive and cannot be patented. For those reasons, there is little interest in either pharmaceutical companies of prescription drugs or OTCs (over-the-counter-drugs) to promote magnesium. However, knowledgeable doctors and health practitioners often do recommend taking a magnesium supplement for specific conditions such as if the person had a stroke or is suffering headaches. But is it not best to avoid health problems before they occur?

Magnesium works ideally with hydrogen peroxide for therapeutic benefits but for protecting and restoring natural wellness. Magnesium should definitely be on your personal health and wellness protocol list.

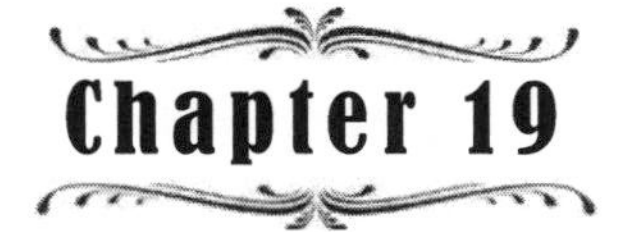

Chapter 19

Single Supplement Mega-Dosing?

How many blogs, TV advertisements and websites claim that you only need to buy their particular product and take large amounts of it in radical mega- dosing you will be cured of every disease, lose weight, become beautiful, and sleep wonderfully?

The majority of alternative healthcare and personal wellness books ultimately reach the shallow and wrong advice of urging you to mega-dose on the single pill, liquid or other supplement the book is about.

It might be urging you to eat massive amounts of wheat grass, kelp or drink gallons of green tea. Or claim that huge levels of calcium, B-12 or Vitamin E or C can prevent all illness and cure all diseases. Or the book might claim that all you need is huge daily amounts of colloidal silver or shark cartilage, some berry that grows in Japan or some root from China and you will be the perfect weight, be immunity from all illness, and cured of cancer, Alzheimer's, HIV/AIDS, and every other possible disease and failing organ. Is one the claimed cure-all health supplement fulvic acid? An amino acid or herb? Or maybe to buy a complex ozone machine, electro-magnetic field generator, or to wear many magnets all over your body.

Such books, blogs, websites, television and radio ads, and magazine ads come out by the tens of thousands a year. Many people read or hear these and believe these claims and sales pitches because they want to believe.

Which one of those single mega-dozing choices it correct? Which one is the perfect preventative and curative self-care choice to make for singular and massive daily mega-dozing?

The answer is none. The human body does not work that way. While such mega-dosing may show positive effects at first due resolving a nutritional deficiency, it also will become counter-productive or harmful quickly.

Why?

Balancing is essential in personal wellness and cellular nutrition. Your cellular health and wellness will decline and collapse if you lack essential and sufficient nutrients and oxygen. Consuming radically high levels of one nutrient or health supplement is not the answer.

Eating an organic grown apple in non-commercial farmed land is good for you. But what if that was all you ever ate exclusively? Would it make sense to eat 50, 100, and then 150 apples a day because a book gave you a schedule of how many more apples you should eat with each coming week or month?

At first, due to having eliminated bad food and eating healthy apples instead would show health benefits for some people. After a few weeks you might see so much improvement, that you are praising the "Apple Therapy." But your body is increasingly depleting other vitamins, minerals, amino acids, enzymes, and other essential nutrients your cells and organs need.

The Goal? Maximized Cellular Oxygen & Nutrient Balance

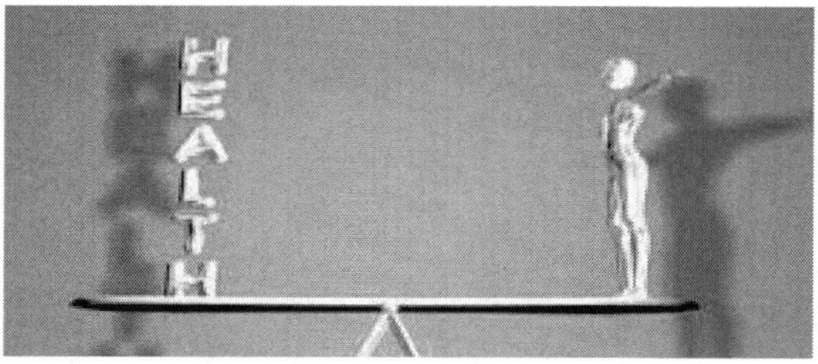

Balance is important in cellular healthcare and wellness plans. In addition to eliminating toxins, harmful chemicals and invasive micro-organisms, viruses, bacterial and fungus from your body and your personal environment and home, give your cellular body and organs all the oxygen and essential nutrients they need. Your body and cells need complete, well-balanced meals. Massively loading up your body with one substance causes imbalance and depletion of other essential vitamins, primary and trace minerals and other vital cellular nutrients.

It has long been known that 1 vitamin can deplete another. Minerals are codependent within the living cellular body for proper functioning. There is a codependency between essential nutrients. Your liver and other organs have to filter and process all cellular nutrients. Single supplement radical mega-dosing floods may overwhelm and come to poison your body, while it is starved and depleted of other essential nutrients.

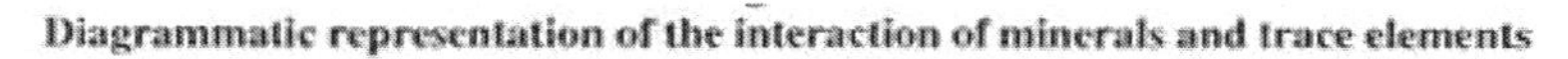
Diagrammatic representation of the interaction of minerals and trace elements

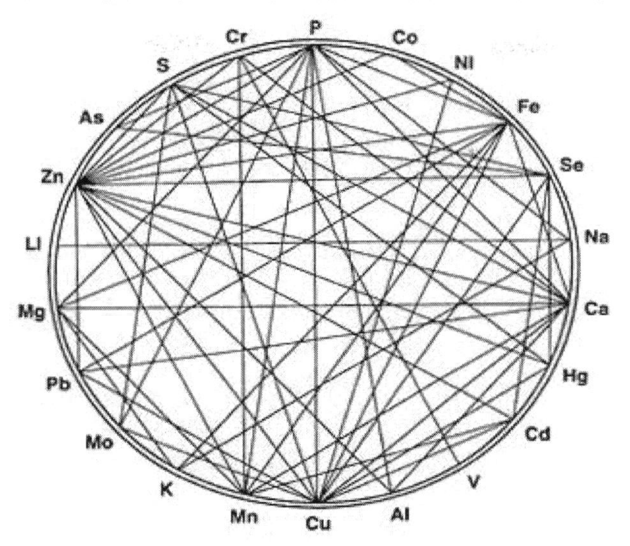

Your inner body functions in the same way as it does outwardly. If you do not eat enough, you will starve and become ill. If you eat too much, you become will gain weight. Oxygenation and cellular nutritional supplementing is the same. Extreme excesses overwork your organs and flood your cellular system preventing natural balancing causing your body to cease to function correctly.

Just as you need sleep, your internal organs need rest too. There also is the question of how do you know precisely how much of each nutritional support your cells and body needs? How do you allow your body to balance itself in essential nutrients and oxygen?

The answer is you don't have to know. Your inner body knows. Your internal body is designed to use and store what it needs and to self-balance – provided it is not overwhelmed.

Allow Your Cellular Body A Day Of Rest

Unless truly necessary otherwise, skip all nutritional supplements 1 day a week. Do not skip prescription medication.

Ideally you would fast one day a week (except for liquids), but that is not essential. Just give your body a day to rest and, in a sense, allow your body, organs, and immune system to sort through the piled up backlog of excessive supplements and distribute all cellular needs through your body.

The fact is that your whole body needs a fully sufficient – but not overly excessive – supply of oxygen and cellular nutrients. Chapter 9 and Chapter 10 presents many different ways to super-oxygenation and promote true wellness body by using 35% food grade hydrogen peroxide.

While massive single substance mega-dosing may seem to offer initial positive benefits, doing so increasingly puts your body out of balance in relation to other vitamins, minerals and essential nutrients. Your cellular body needs oxygenation and all essential substances, but in at balanced, non-excessive levels.

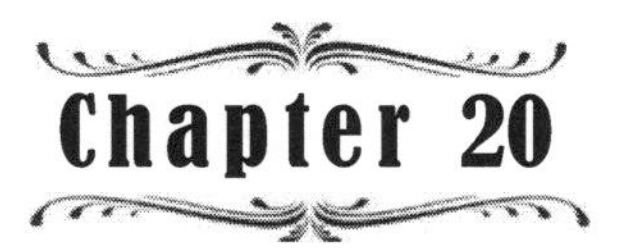

Chapter 20

Natural Sea Salt

Sea salt is the easiest way to spice up your diet and to benefit your health at the same time. Sea salt also will reduce your salt intake as sea salts tend to taste saltier.

Salt is the only spice necessary for life. Salt is the most often used seasoning for food. Those who have not experienced replacing processed "table salt" with organic sea salts do not realize that like all spices, different salts provide different flavors. The selection of salt is a critical decision to all the world's great chefs and finest restaurants.

The health benefits of sea salts are found both in their high mineral content (grocery store salt is devoid of minerals and their high sodium to chloride ratio). The most fundamental and highly used spice is salt. While excessive salt intake is harmful, depletion of salt is ultimately lethal. Salt is a natural adversary to many fungus, bacteria, and viruses. Our bodies are dependent upon an intake of a sufficient but not excessive intake of salt.

Gourmet salts are among the secret ingredients of the finest restaurants. They will pay as much as $50 per pound or more for special sea salts rather than pennies for processed grocery store salt. Each salt has its unique taste due to its unique mix of minerals and the complex variations of salt crystals. Until you try sea salts, you probably believe all salt tastes the same, but this is very inaccurate.

Salt, the most commonly used of all seasonings, is defined by its contents. For sea salts this includes various ratios of minerals and various ratios of the remnants of the micro sea life that lived and died in the water. All life on earth is dependent upon the smallest creatures of the sea. The complex beneficial organic interactions occur within those tiny creatures upon minerals and amino acids, which remain within the sea salt from their remains. This also is lacking in common table salt.

It takes less sea salt for the same level of saltiness as generic table salt thus preventing excessive salt intake. The saltier taste helps you avoid excessive salt intake. Sea salts contain dozens of trace minerals necessary for life. Processed salt does not. Most table salt is surface mined from large salt flats. Their minerals were leached out long ago.

Refined salt is devoid of all minerals and complex molecular structures – unique to each source of the sea salt. "Grocery store" sea salt is the by-product of desalination plants. There are MANY reasons NOT to use cheap generic sea salt found in grocery stores for this reason. First, this salt tends to be highly contaminated due to the water sources used for desalination factories. The process also strips away most mineral content and the heat process used in desalination destroys the complex micro-structures of sea salt and salt water.

You may find this difficult to believe until you experience fine sea salts, but sea salt can become somewhat addictive and it is common for people to carry it in their purses or little containers for when they go restaurant dining. Many natural minerals have their unique taste. Vitamin/mineral pills are usually coated to block any taste so many people believe that minerals are tasteless. The complex subtle ratios and mixes within sea salt and within each salt granule make it impossible to artificially duplicate. What seasoning is more critical in cooking than salt?

Those who learn to enjoy gourmet cooking or just want variety in their meals know the importance of their selections of specialty and imported sea salt for each specific dish they are preparing. A little goes a long way.

Among the finest chefs and restaurants, they realize that diversity in salt selection also prevents all their food from tasting the same. Fine Sea Salts are their secret ingredient and why their gourmet meals have so taste better taste and are more flavorful – though seemingly the ingredients are the same as typical restaurants.

Documented medical studies have shown enormous health benefits resulting from changing from processed table salt to sea salt. This foremost is due to increasing mineral intake and reducing sodium chloride intake.

However, some also believe some sea salts are naturally ionized, therefore assisting to maintaining and restoring the ionic and magnetic field within cell structures of the human body due to dramatic reduction in the earth's magnetic fields.

Many people will add some salt (not much) to water they drink for this reason and medical studies have shown health benefits in doing so. It can remove bitterness from coffee. Salt is anti-bacterial. Salt is the most ancient preservative for that reason.

You will love how it improves the taste of your food. You will enjoy actually chewing your food, rather than just wolfing it down quickly. People who eat slower also tend to eat less. Your intake of sodium chloride will be reduced, If you enjoy your meals more it is likely you will still desire for high calorie, low health value sweets and snacks. At the same time your cellular body is receiving critical trace minerals that were previously lacking in your food.

Sea salt will go a long way and can be used in place of table salt for all cooking. For cooking, try many different kinds. Each adds different flavor to your food and will have various ratios of trace minerals. As a result, you will come to reduce the amount of salt of you use. At the same time your cells and organs are receiving the benefits of the all essential trace minerals.

Best natural sea salt? *It is found in a mountain!*

Himalayan Pink Mountain Salt

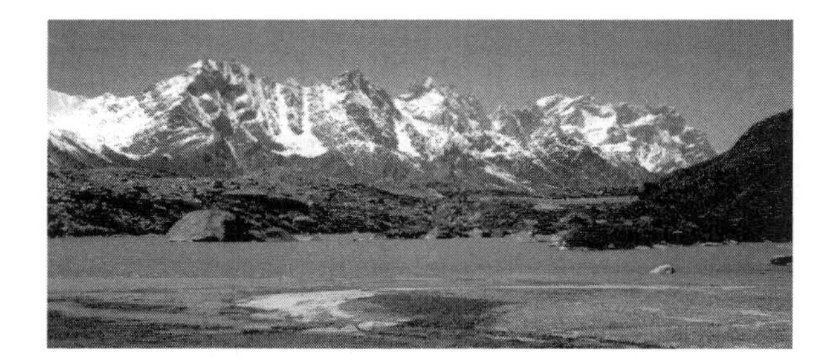

The ancient salt of the Himalayan Mountains contains millions of years of accumulation of essential trace minerals that you cannot obtain in your food. Switching from processed table salt to using Himalayan salt is one source to provide your cells vital trace minerals lacking in food.

Because the source is from deep within the Himalayan Mountain range where it has been safety trapped for hundreds of millions of years; it has never been exposed to any modern chemicals, toxins, and radiation sources – making it the purest of all salt – processed or sea salt. Because it is trapped within the mountains themselves, the minerals have not been leached out – making it the highest diverse ratio of minerals of unique decomposed ancient organic structures of any sea salt; offering unique health benefits and while at the same time offering a subtle and unique taste.

For the best gourmet and cook salt as per mineral content most agree on Himalayan salt. Himalayan salt is a very ancient salt mined from mountains of Tibet. For the known history of Tibet, they have followed salt shafts deeper and deeper into the Himalayan Mountains. For millenniums, Himalayan Mountain Sea Salt has been considered to have mystical properties among Tibetan.

Himalayan Mountain salt is still mined, transported by hand and naturally sundried in the same manner for over 2000 years.

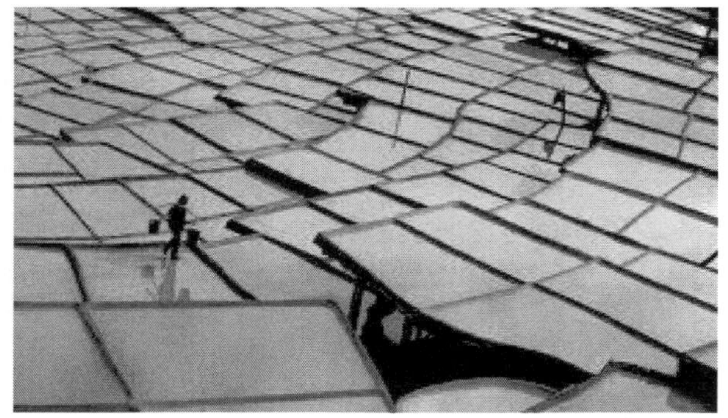

The health benefits of its unique structure had been long recognized.

This is due to how extremely ancient the salt is. Since the ancient ocean dried to form a salt bed many hundreds of feet deep, the entire area was pushed up to make the highest mountain range in the world, with two earth crust plates pushing one over the other across hundreds of millions of years – also then covering over the sea bed with rock. Originating from this ancient ocean, possibly at the origins of life itself the endless movement of the earth's crust eventually pushed this extremely ancient sea salt bed into the Himalayan Mountain range bordering Tibet and Pakistan

Best Sea Salt for Mineral Soak Bathing?

Dead Sea Salt

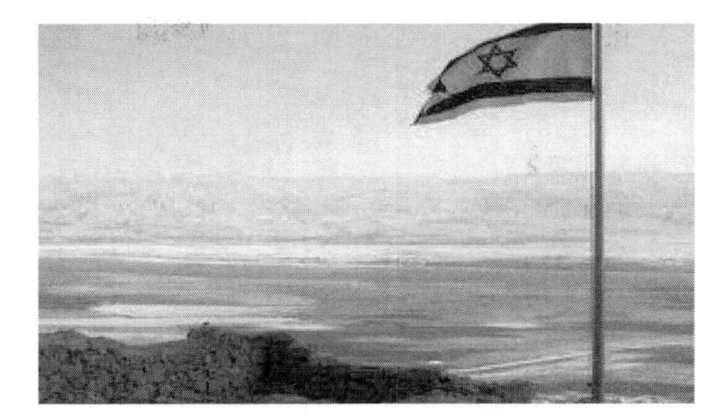

The best sea salt for bathing is Dead Sea Salt from Israel. Himalayan salt would also be excellent, but would stain your tub.

In the Roman Era the Nile River and delta was lush due to the climate being wetter. Annually the Nile would flood, renewing the soil with mineral nutrients. The Roman soldier's diet was mostly grain: wheat, barley, and oats, spelt and rye from the Nile Region, not meat or crops from farmed land in Italy. Although not understanding nutrient theory, they learned their Legions could march further and fight harder on a diet of "Roman Meal" from that region of the world.

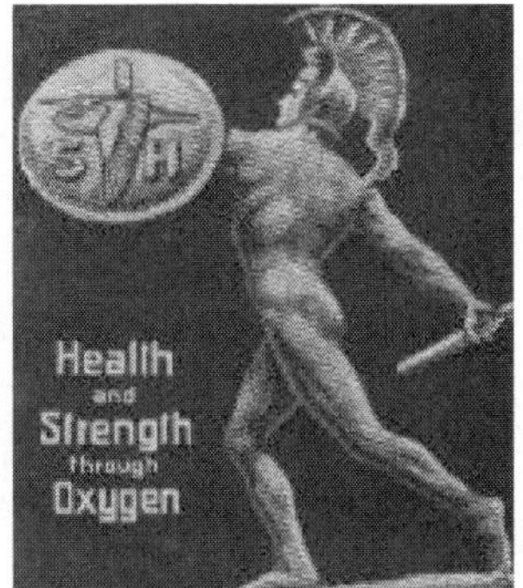

High in minerals that washed off the highly fertile surrounding ancient lands, the mineral content of Dead Sea Salt is very high. The health benefits of the mineral rich soil of this region in the past were so recognized that the Romans believed feeding their legions with wheat and barley from this region was an absolute necessity for the stamina of Roman Legionnaires. This is primary reason why they considered the region of such great strategic importance.

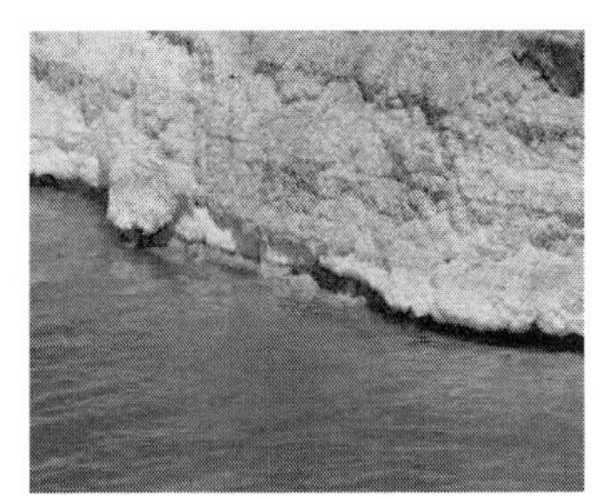

Israeli Dead Sea Salt is produced by natural solar drying waters of the ancient waters of the Dead Sea.

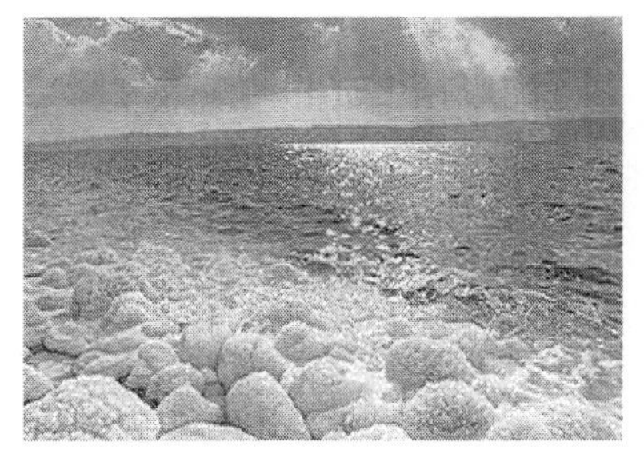

Bathing in the Dead Sea for health benefits has been practiced for centuries and the Dead Sea is the saltiest water in the world.

However, not all Dead Sea salt is suitable for the kitchen so be cautious. Some that is ideally suited for mineral soaking your body tastes absolutely horrible. For the kitchen you should be careful to buy Dead Sea Salt specific for cooking. All gourmet Dead Sea salt is suitable for body mineral soaking.

Millions of people worldwide use fine ground Dead Sea salt in their salt shakers and cooking. It also is very popular for spas and hot tubs.

Hint For Hot Tub Owners

The Dead Sea is a popular center for wellness and health today. You can bathe your skin in mineral rich Dead Sea salt by adding it to your hot tub. Every time you soak in your hot tub you are feeding your body essential trace minerals. Salt is also powerful biocide that will help keep your hot tub clean and free of most biological mirco-organism. Dead Sea salt has the following benefits:

Rheumatologic Conditions – Dead Sea salts can be effective in balneotherapy of rheumatoid arthritis, psoriatic arthritis, and osteoarthritis. The minerals are absorbed while soaking, stimulating blood circulation.

Common skin ailments – Research has demonstrated that skin disorders such as acne and psoriasis are relieved by regular soaking in water with added Dead Sea salt. The National Psoriasis Foundation recommends Dead Sea and Dead Sea salts as effective treatments for psoriasis.

One study concluded that the high concentration of magnesium in Dead Sea salt was instrumental in improving skin hydration and reducing inflammation.

Allergies – The high concentration of trace minerals and magnesium in the Dead Sea salt can relieve allergic reactions by cleansing and detoxifying.

Skin aging – Further research into Dead Sea salt benefits has shown a 40% reduction in the depth of wrinkling.

HOW TO CONSIDER HEALTH & WELLNESS?

> You must learn a new way to think before you can master a new way to be.
>
> Marianne Williamson

Is this information relevant to you? Many tell themselves, "I do not have those health issues. I am healthy so this is not relevant to me."

In fact, all of this information is relevant to you. Remember the old saying: "An ounce of prevention is worth a pound of cure." It is far easier to avoid a health crisis or problem than to cure it.

If you do have a serious adverse medical condition, your body's immune system may already be severely weakened – and busy trying to cure you of the unknown condition. You possibly are far more susceptible to additional health issues or may even come to face with a growing catastrophic health collapse.

Easy changes in your choices can cause decisive improvements in your overall physical and mental health and wellness. As the example of this chapter, merely changing what salt you use for your food can make the difference of whether your cellular body receives any trace minerals or is completely trace mineral depleted. It is a myth that personal health care is difficult, expensive and time consuming. But it also is untrue when someone says everything will take care of itself. Only you can take care of your cellular body and wellbeing.

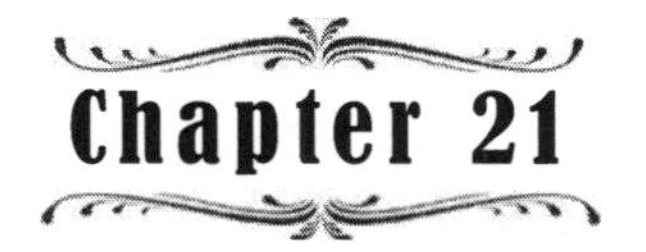

Chapter 21

Storage of Hydrogen Peroxide

35% food grade hydrogen peroxide must be stored in the dark and in a cool location. UV light causes 35% food grade hydrogen peroxide to decompose.

CAUTION – PERSONAL SAFETY:

Wear plastic gloves and safety goggles when adding 35% food grade hydrogen peroxide to the water as it can splash or spill. You simply add the hydrogen peroxide to the water and no special injection system is necessary.

STORE SAFELY:

Do not store 35% food grade hydrogen peroxide in a freezer. While storage in a refrigerator is ideal, a cool totally dark location is acceptable. Remember to slightly loosen the cap as true 35% food grade hydrogen peroxide has no stabilizing chemicals and will gradually swell the bottle.

It is important to safeguard concentrated hydrogen peroxide from children and adults who are not competent enough to not consume substances they do not know what they are.

STORE HYDROGEN PEROXIDE IN THE DARK

35% food grade hydrogen peroxide rapidly decomposes in photo-reaction to U.V. light. This will cause the hydrogen peroxide to weaken in concentration and will cause the bottle to expand and possibly burst.

Slightly loosening the cap (slightly) to allow for any gas build up to bleed off rather than burst the bottle in which it is stored for an extended period. Storing in the dark means total darkness (though the brief refrigerator light when open or while mixing under kitchen light is acceptable as is when you are pouring or using it.)

DO NOT STORE IN FREEZER

There is a false view commonly taken that food grade hydrogen peroxide should be stored in the freezer. If 35% food grade hydrogen peroxide is frozen at too cold a temperature, it will separate (decompose) as the 65% of it that is water and the 35% food grade hydrogen peroxide freeze at different temperatures. Do not store 35% food grade hydrogen peroxide in a freezer.

STORE IN REFRIGERATOR IF PRACTICAL & SAFE

Small bottles of hydrogen peroxide are best stored in a refrigerator as it is cold and dark. However, this is only the case if this is hydrogen peroxide is not accessible to children or incompetent adults. Otherwise, simply store hydrogen peroxide in any cool, dark location. Extra bottles are best stored in their box, the bottle upright, and the slightly loosened the cap.

DO NOT STORE IN A GLASS CONTAINER

Laboratories prefer chemicals in glass containers so they do not have to remember what chemicals are suited for plastic and which ones are not. They also know to exercise great care in handling chemical containers.

It is always possible a container will slip out of someone's hand or accidently knocked of a kitchen counter. Someone else might move it and drop it. This would splash the hydrogen peroxide along with broken glass. The container you used would not contain safety information and possibly would not even advise what it is it to others.

Other than small dropper bottles that people commonly use for counting drops, do not store your hydrogen peroxide in glass containers.

HOW LONG CAN HYDROGEN PEROXIDE BE STORED?

At temperatures of 70 degrees or lower (but not much below freezing), 35% food grade hydrogen peroxide will on average decompose (lose strength) at a rate of less than 1% per month. Higher temperature will increase decomposition, but not significantly unless the temperature is well over 80 degrees. Do not store 35% food grade hydrogen peroxide near a heat source such as hot water heater. The colder it is stored the slower in decomposes.

Properly stored, 35% food grade hydrogen peroxide can be stored for a long time. Given its anti-bacterial and anti-fungal nature, 35% food grade hydrogen peroxide will not spoil. The primary cause of 35% food grade hydrogen peroxide losing its potency is prolonged exposure to UV light from any source. It is very important to store 35% food grade hydrogen peroxide in the dark.

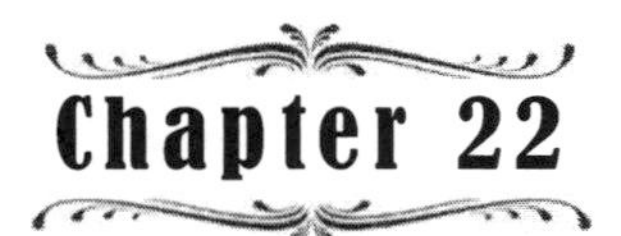

Chapter 22

So Many Uses Of Hydrogen Peroxide

A special thank you to those individuals and organizations that provided this information.

There are so many beneficial and wellness usages of 35% food grade hydrogen peroxide. Here are some of the most common and best uses of 35% food grade hydrogen peroxide.

INTERNAL USAGE (Read warnings below first)

Safe Usage level: 4 to 8 drops per 8 ounces of distilled or filtered water between meals, 2 to 3 times a day, 5 to 6 days a week. You should start at a lower rather than higher level. NEVER consume hydrogen peroxide in concentrated form. It MUST be HIGHLY diluted first.

For health and wellness therapy, oral usage and super-oxygenation therapy, See Chapter 10, which involves higher usage levels.

KEEP OUT OF YOUR EYES.

Hydrogen peroxide can cause severe eye damage.

NEVER inject 35% food grade hydrogen peroxide by needle or other means into your body.

HIGHER LEVEL USAGE: Any higher concentration levels of 35% food grade hydrogen peroxide internal usage should be approached gradually. Excessive levels can be harmful.

WARNING SIGNS OF EXCESSIVE USAGE:

35% food grade hydrogen peroxide has a distinct taste to it. However, if there is any stinging sensation in the mouth the level is too high. If there is any internal sense of stinging or stomach pain, drink as much water as possible and seek immediate emergency medical attention.

Never induce vomiting as this can cause throat and lung damage.

Occasionally people who use 35% food grade hydrogen peroxide for the first time will report diarrhea. This is not uncommon and should end soon. This is due to the body flushing out waste materials. Serious stomach pain, however, is a serious warning sign of excessive concentration and should be taken seriously.

If the stomach pain is intense drink as much water as you can. If this does not cause prompt ending of the stomach pain, seek immediate emergency medical care.

If you are gradually increasing levels of 35% food grade hydrogen peroxide consumption across a period of time, warning signs that the levels are becoming excessive are a sensation of stomach gas or blood shot eyes. You should discontinue usage for a day or two, and then resume at a lower level of concentration.

Swimming Pool and Hot Tub usage:

Getting started – Many recommend shocking your pool or tub to start using hydrogen peroxide. To "SHOCK" your pool or hot tub, a relatively high level is used at a ratio of 1 cup for every 250 gallons.

Do not run your pump continuously. Rather, run it only long enough to circulate the water and then turn off the pump. Ideally, you should add the 35% food grade hydrogen peroxide at sunset and allow the water to sit 24 hours before turning the pump back on. The tub or pool may be used afterwards. It is not necessary to shock your pool or hot tub if you are starting with fresh water. 35% food grade hydrogen peroxide will not adversely interact with other pool chemicals.

POOL AND HOT TUB MAINTENANCE:

This depends on the water source and the amount of organic materials that enter the water (dust, leaves, number of people using the pool etc.) If you are starting with new water, a good starting point is 1 cup of 35% food grade hydrogen peroxide for every 500 gallons of water. 35% food grade hydrogen peroxide interacts with and oxidizes organic materials and decomposes with UV light. This is a reason that 35% food grade hydrogen peroxide must be added time to time to maintain its level in the water. There is no danger of 35% food grade hydrogen peroxide forming dangerous residual chemicals.

TEST STRIPS: There are test strips to measure the PPM concentration of hydrogen peroxide in pool and spa water. Ideally, keep the concentration level measuring between 500 and 1000 ppm. Test strips can be found for such testing.

CHECK YOUR FILTERS OFTEN: As with any pool or hot tub with a filtration system, regularly check your filter(s) as clogged filters will damage some pumping systems.

WASH AND PRESERVE FRESH FRUIT AND VEGETABLES:

Food spoilage and food poisoning both are the result of the growth of microorganisms in fresh cut fruits and vegetables. Increasingly, food packers have begun switching to use of hydrogen peroxide as a disinfecting agent due to the safety issues of using chlorine. 35% food grade hydrogen peroxide is a powerful anti-microbial which may be used not only for washing fruits and vegetables free of pesticides and other contaminants present, but also to extend the shelf life of these fresh products and elimination of the microorganisms delays spoilage.

If you are tired of how quickly fresh produce spoils even if refrigerated, washing vegetables in a 35% food grade hydrogen peroxide solution will cure both problems without any of the toxic effects of chlorine. Dilution ratio: 1/8 cup 35% food grade hydrogen peroxide per 1-gallon water.

TIRED OF LETTUCE GOING BAD AFTER YOU START TO USE IT?

Ever notice that after you open a head of lettuce, it starts to go bad within hours – turning brown? This is due to invasion of micro-organisms by touching and handling. Dilution: If you keep a gallon jug with 1/2 ounce 35% food grade hydrogen peroxide to the gallon and rinse the head off before putting it in a sealed plastic container (shake off the excess diluted 35% food grade hydrogen peroxide solution first) and it will last longer before it turns.

HAND WASH:

Many medical experts agree that most colds and the flu are not passed in the air, but through the hands. You shake hands with other people, touch where they touched and whether in eating, rubbing your nose, smoking a cigarette, chewing your fingernails, etc. – pass this on to yourself via your hands. Experts agree that washing your hands often is the best way to reduce catching many diseases.

Dilution: To make a good hand wash, use 1 ounce per 1 pint *(2 cups)* 35% 35% food grade hydrogen peroxide. You also may add hand soap to a hand soap pump bottle. Now, you also are using a powerful antiseptic.

TO PRESERVE MEAT:

The primary cause of meat spoilage is micro-organisms. Meat packers learned long ago that if they can keep meat from being touched it will not spoil for months. Professional butchers never touch the meat directly if cutting it and will frequently dip their knives in sterilizing solution to avoid contaminating the meat.

If you are tired of your meat spoiling within a day or two of arriving from the grocery *store (cutters in grocery stores tend not to follow these standards)*, wash fresh meat *(beef, poultry and pork – but not hamburger or ground meat)* in an 35% food grade hydrogen peroxide solution and put it in a zip-lock bag. It will then last for weeks instead of days. Dilution: Same as vegetables and fruit above.

HOUSE & GARDEN PLANTS:

To watch your plants grow and become healthy add a few drops of food grade hydrogen peroxide per gallon of water.

Plants thrive with 35% food grade hydrogen peroxide and it benefits them in two ways. First, it oxygenates the soil. Second, it kills micro-organisms, fungus and bacteria harmful to plants. It will not harm worms due to the dilution. Houseplants and gardens thrive with 35% food grade hydrogen peroxide supplementing and an increasing number of commercial farmers using 35% food grade hydrogen peroxide.

Dilution ratio for plants: Put 1/2 ounce 35% food grade per gallon water for plant watering and for water to soak seeds for sprouting.

Sprouting needs: Add 1 ounce of 3% hydrogen peroxide to one pint of water and soak the seeds overnight. Add the same amount of hydrogen peroxide each time you rinse the seeds.

KITCHEN, BATHROOM AND GENERAL SANITIZING:

Chlorine, bleach, and ammonia are very toxic both in liquid form and the fumes they cause. 35% food grade hydrogen peroxide is the safe and wise alternative.

Use it to wipe down kitchen counters, to mop the floor and particularly wipe down the refrigerator interior (kills the organisms leading to spoilage.) It will sterilize the toilet bowl. Bathrooms tend to collect many micro-organisms so wipe the bathroom down with it as well. Wipe out the children's lunch box to eliminate odors. Hydrogen Peroxide is great for eliminating kitchen odors. Dilution ratio: 1 cup 35% food grade hydrogen peroxide per 1 gallon water. Note: the dilute ion ratio of 1 ounce per 1 quart is good for face wash water, and good to reduce acne as well. But do not use around your eyes any stronger than this and if in doubt, dilute further.

CLOTHING/LAUNDRY:

35% food grade hydrogen peroxide is a safe alternative to harmful bleach. The finest clothing manufacturers use 35% food grade hydrogen peroxide, not bleach, as their whitening agent. Bleach residual against your skin is harmful to you skin and chloride vapor in the air is very harmful to health. Replace bleach with 35% food grade hydrogen peroxide.

<u>But also remember hydrogen peroxide has a bleaching effect on fabric.</u>

Tip: Pillows and pillowcases are atrocious for gathering micro-pests. Every month or so you should rotate the pillows you sleep on. Remove the pillowcase and seal the old one in a black plastic trash bag and leave it in the sun (if possible). At the end of the month, all the mites, fungus, bacteria and other microorganisms are gone. Rotate your pillows this way. The only alternative is to wash in a 35% food grade hydrogen peroxide solution *(if pillow is washable and most actually are).*

DILUTION FOR LAUNDRY:

½ cup of 35% food grade hydrogen peroxide per wash load. You may increase this amount for a stronger bleaching effect on whites if you wish. 35% food grade hydrogen peroxide will also kill the millions of micro-mites and pests that gather in bedding. Pay particular attention to pillowcases.

DILUTION FOR DISHWASHER:

½ cup 35% food grade hydrogen peroxide into the dishwasher and the dishes will sparkle and are sanitized. Or use 1 ounce per gallon sink water if you wash your dishes in the sink.

FOR BATH WATER:

Add 2 cups of 35% food grade hydrogen peroxide to your tub after you fill it. Soak for 10 to 15 minutes. Do not shampoo your hair as the hydrogen peroxide may lighten your hair. You may refresh the tub with hot water to keep it comfortable.

For a fabulous bath soak, add the sea salt *(1-2 cups)* and Epson salt **(1/4th to ½ pound).** Shower before exiting tub.

Caution: This will relax your muscles. Be careful not to fall asleep and be careful getting out of the tub. This would be excellent prior to a mid- day nap or just before bedtime.

FOR PET'S BATH WATER:

For small animals (dogs and cats) use 1 ounce 35% hydrogen peroxide to 1-gallon water for their bath water.

FOR PETS DRINKING WATER:

For drinking water, the dilution should be no stronger than 4 drops 35% food grade hydrogen peroxide per 1 gallon of water. Remember to keep your pet's bedding clean. 35% food grade hydrogen peroxide is a great sterilizing agent. Wash a cat litter box with the 35% food grade hydrogen peroxide kitchen cleaning mix described above and odors are gone – and are not replaced with horrible bleach smells.

AQUARIUM CLEAN-UP:

Never use 35% food grade hydrogen peroxide for aquarium water with the fish still in it as some species of fish are very chemical specific in vulnerability. However, 35% food grade hydrogen peroxide can be used for aquarium clean up (with the fish out) and would kill the micro-organisms that make the rocks and decorations in an aquarium stink.

After using the 35% food grade hydrogen peroxide cleaning solution, use 2 ounces of 35% food grade hydrogen peroxide per gallon of water and let it soak a while. Then rinse again with fresh water. Odors and micro-organisms are gone. As an aquarium does not have the natural self-cleaning ability as rivers, lakes, and oceans do; you should periodically not only clean, but also sterilize your aquarium.

FOR FEET:

Feet get quite the abuse being trapped in the same shoes day after day – for which the micro-pest level becomes high. For a good foot soak, add 2 ounces 35% hydrogen peroxide to 1 of gallon water. This also will help to avoid foot problems before they start. This will prevent athlete's foot and will treat it with repeated foot soaks.

MOUTHWASH:

This level is too high for internal consumption. Do not swallow. This not only kills the bacteria that causes bad breathe and goes a long way to preventing tooth decay, it also has a whitening effect. Dilute 35% food grade hydrogen peroxide on a 1-16 ratio *(1 part 35% food grade hydrogen peroxide to 16 parts water)*. Do not use as a mouthwash in higher concentration. *(This is one ounce per 1 pint or 2 cups of water)*.

You can mix this up in advance in and leave the bottle under the bathroom counter. Be certain to mark it with a warning and secure it if there are children in your home. The contents will remain sterile due to the sterilizing effect of 35% food grade hydrogen peroxide. This is 10 times as effective as typical alcohol based mouth wash. Swish it around in your mouth for 1-2 minutes before brushing. Do not exceed the concentration. See Chapter 10 for oxygenation by mouth.

WARNINGS ABOUT INTERNAL USAGE:

The FDA has not approved of any medical application or internal usage of hydrogen peroxide. Hydrogen peroxide should never be used for any medical purpose and never ingested *(swallowed)* unless is it greatly reduced.

You should never inject hydrogen peroxide in any concentration into your blood stream and doing so may result in permanent injury or death.

Such direct injection into the blood stream should only be administered by a licensed doctor and then it would be administered in a highly diluted form at a very slow and regulated rate.

Hydrogen peroxide at any concentration level should never be used as eyewash, for cleaning ears or as a nasal spray.

There is no established level of safe oral ingesting of hydrogen peroxide, though it has been used in 3% concentration as mouthwash for decades *(though not to be swallowed at the level).* Any oral consumption of any hydrogen peroxide should only be considered if it is highly diluted.

You should never inject hydrogen peroxide in any concentration into your blood stream yourself. Doing so yourself may cause permanent injury or death. Such direct injection should only be administered by a licensed doctor or qualified health care profession - and then it would only be administered in a very highly diluted form. Hydrogen peroxide at any concentration level should never be used for eyewash, for cleaning ears, or as a nasal spray.

Hydrogen peroxide should never be self-administered in a manner that directly injects or puts hydrogen peroxide into the blood stream unless done by a fully qualified and licensed healthcare professional. Doing so yourself will likely result in permanent injury or death.

Chapters 9 & 10 presented using 35% food grade hydrogen peroxide for oxygenation and wellness therapy.

Chapter 23

Personal Wellness Checklist

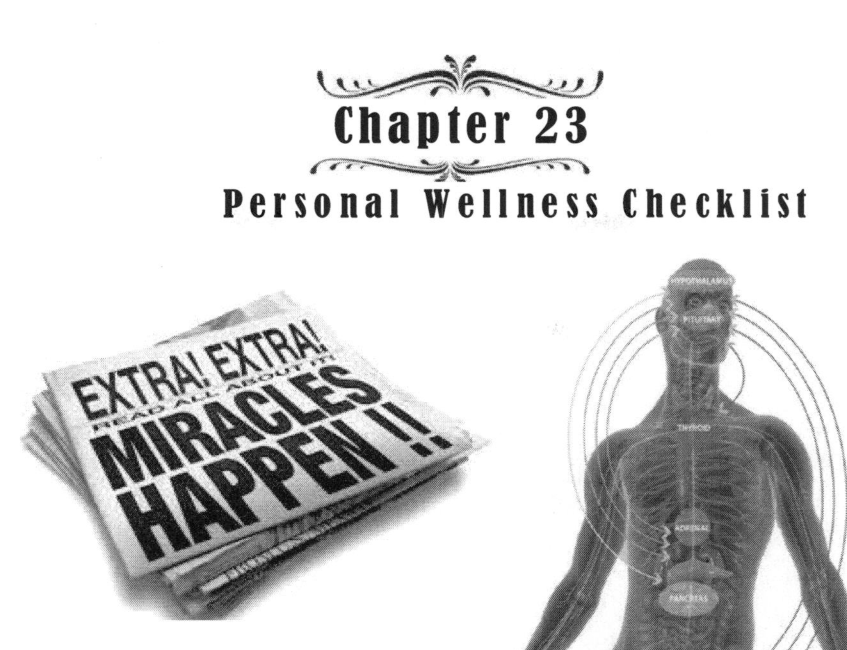

There are many simple steps to complete cellular health for physical whole body wellness. This chapter provides you with easy guidelines and specific actions that you can use in your daily life.

It may surprise you how easy and inexpensive establishing and following your personal health and wellness protocol is. While I would hope you will follow all of these, any of these will improve your health and, residually, then your life. If you just remember to air out our house and not deplete the oxygen by candles, gas stoves and other oxygen depletion sources the book was well worth reading.

What follows in this chapter is a checklist for you to review and evaluate.

Consider 35% food grade hydrogen peroxide internal usage therapy, not exceeding safe levels, for blood oxygenation and purifying.

Replace your cleaning chemicals with 35% food grade hydrogen peroxide.

Replace table salt with sea salt. The best is Himalayan salt. But any non-processed true white sea salt is excellent.

Avoid synthetic clothes.

At least once a week soak in your bathtub with hydrogen peroxide, magnesium (Epson salt) and natural sea salt. *See Chapter 9 or Chapter 21.* Add 2 cups of 35% food grade hydrogen peroxide to your tub after you fill it. Add the sea salt (1-2 cups) and Epson salt ($1/4^{th}$ to one-half pound) when you start to fill the tub so it can dissolve.

Take a liquid trace mineral supplement. Insure that you take a sufficient level of vitamins and minerals.

If you have allergies, and if your budget allows for it, eliminate carpeting, particularly from your bedroom. If not, regularly vacuum it with a HEPA filter vacuum cleaner.

Cease using chlorine and bromine in your pool and/or hot tub. Do not use bleach and chlorine for cleaning. Use 35% food grade hydrogen peroxide that has been diluted.

Do not use bug bombs in your home. Limit pesticide usage in your home. The best pest control is a clean kitchen. Using powered boric acid will address most insect problems.

Eliminate processed sugar and bleached flour as much as comfortable from your diet.

Go through your house to find all chemicals that you use. Read the warnings. If a chemical product label warns not to breathe the fumes stop using it if possible. Make certain the cap is closed tightly. When you must use it have doors and windows open with a fan blowing outward.

Buy a supply of latex free gloves to wear when using harsh chemicals. Your skin is porous.

Use a HEPA rated vacuum cleaner.

Put a HEPA rated air filter machine at least in your bedroom. They are inexpensive at hardware stores or look online. You do not want filters with Febreze ™ and all products that "smell" such as "air fresheners" and scented candles. If you must have scented air, use natural herbs and spices.

Cook foods and meat at less than 300 degrees, but for a sufficient time. Avoid boiling vegetables.

Frequently air out your house; especially if you have synthetic furniture and drapery.

Add window locks that allow you to have your windows partially open at least part of the day and definitely allow your bedroom window to be cracked open at night. These locks are inexpensive. Ask for them at any hardware store. They allow you to have your window partially open while still preventing anyone entering. Definitely install window locks for personal safety to allow cracking the windows open, while not enough for anyone to enter for your personal safety.

Having a fresh air flow in your bedroom is particularly critical if you have gas heat. Ventilate your house while using a gas stove or oven.

Add a couple of drops of 35% food grade hydrogen peroxide to your pets and plants water.

If your budget allows add a **whole-house water filtration system.** If not, definitely filter both your drinking and cooking water.

Knowledge sharing:

If you have creative or useful suggestions for this chapter, please email those to me at:

PowerOfHydrogenPeroxide@gmail.com
(Put in subject line: "Attn Mary")

The next 3 chapters bring the whole picture together.

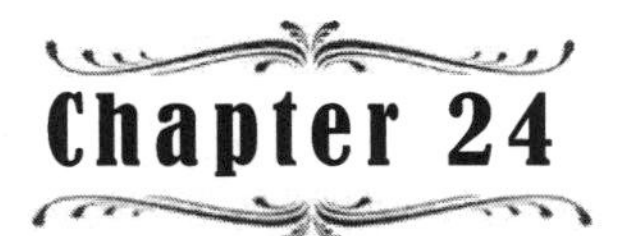

Chapter 24

Listen to Your Cellular Body

> You have 75 Trillion Cells. You create 10 million cells per second. Your job is simple: Give them what they need.

Your body has 75 TRILION cells.

Ponder of that for a moment. 75 TRILLION living breathing cells.

Is the human body a super colony of an incredible collective intelligence? Or only a mindless organic machine? I refer to this subject as "Organic Metaphysics," but will not go into great detail in this book.

The cells of your body are a living collective colony of living and thinking organisms that in fact do communicate with each other and you in many ways. They tell you when your body is thirsty and hungry. They tell you when they are running out of energy. They tell you when they are tired and warn of dangers by touch and smell.

A complex and challenging question is if a person catches a cold, is it the cold that causes your temperature to go up, causes the other symptoms and for you to be weak and tired? Or is your body doing those things in self-defense until it figures out how to destroy the millions of invasive virus of that cold?

Is it your cellular body that raises your body temperature - while convincing you to also put on a blanket - and makes you tired and in bed. Does your cellular body do this so it can maximize their energy levels by heat and have the heat expand your blood vessels for maximum blood flow; thus allowing them better access and more oxygen and nutrients as they study, isolate, attack and destroy the invasive virus?

Did your cellular body make you feel tired and put you in bed to allow devoting all their efforts towards defeating that cold? Did your cellular body make you sweat so your largest organ that you have – your skin –is in the battle by expelling toxins and dead virus cells? Does your cellular body make you cough to expel the virus out of your lungs and make your nose runny also to expel the virus?

Your cellular body does communicate to you. But do you listen?

In this book I avoided the hundreds of personal anecdotal accounts of others and myself as there is reason to question their accuracy. But I will inject one here that occurred while I was reviewing a chapter of this book.

Visiting a friend who is very energy efficiency conscious for the weekend, we had returned to her house that is perfectly sealed for energy efficiency. I decided to work on one chapter of this book while she said she would "heat up the house" as it was quite cold out and she turns down the thermostat when leaving.

As I sat at the desk in the guest bedroom, within 45 minutes I felt extremely tired and could not focus. So tired, all I wanted to do was lay my head on the desk not even wanting to take the time to go to the bed.

But I know this is not typical for me. I KNEW my body was trying to put me to sleep for a reason. So I explored and quickly found the reason. My friend was trying to quickly heat the house by using her gas oven with the oven door open. That explained why my body was trying to shut me down mentally and physically by putting me to sleep. The amount of oxygen in the air was rapidly reducing.

Fire burns oxygen very quick. Drop a lite match in an empty bottle and it with be extinguished by lack of oxygen within a couple seconds because it used (burned) away the oxygen. Her oven has rows of gas burns that were rapidly using up the oxygen in her house that is so sealed there was no way for it to be replaced. It this growing oxygen crisis, my cellular body was trying to put me to sleep to minimize the energy I was expending to minimize the need for oxygen. I had heard my body's messaging to me.

The solution was as simple as opening the bedroom window (and explaining to her that the oven was burning up the oxygen.)

This example is not only to stress the importance of fresh air in your home and to warn that candles, the fireplace and gas ovens and stoves when used deplete the air of vital oxygen – so be sure to have a fresh air source. It is also to urge you to LISTEN to what your body is trying to tell you.

If you start to feel exhausted, short of breathe, dizzy, weak or cannot focus, there IS a reason. Do not ignore it. It may be warning you of something VERY serious. For example, an increasing loss of energy, feeling exhausted and lack of stamina can be a warning of an impending heart attack. So LAY OR SIT DOWN. Promptly. Free our mind and relax. Slow down your metabolism and lighten the load on your heart. You should have a doctor check you ASAP. Never ignore your body's attempts to communicate to you.

All the great medical minds from around the world for centuries still cannot cure the common cold. Often all they can do is treat the symptoms to make you comfortable while your immune system and cellular body both best adjust all your body functions to keep you alive, while at the same time figuring out what modern medicine cannot - how to totally destroy the virus.

If you ponder how trillions of cells in your body act in miraculous harmony to destroy the invasive virus, you start to understand a little of how absolutely amazing and brilliant your cellular body is.

Vaccinations work by infecting your body with a weakened form of virus so your body learns how to destroy it. Most diseases can only be cured by your own body, not medicine. Once your body knows how to destroy a particular virus or other invasive micro-organism, almost without exception it will REMEMBER how and will immediately destroy such an invasion. The vaccination served to EDUCATE your cellular body and immune system.

An upset stomach, headache, and any physical pain all is our intelligent body trying to communicate with us.

> Change "I" to "we" to know the real "me."

These are known realities of the super-colony of your cellular body:

- Your cellular body communicates with you.
- Your cellular body is capable of complex learning.
- Your cellular body has highly skilled problem solving skills.

- Your cells share their collectively learned information and pass it to the next generation of cells.

- Your cellular body has a complex memory.

- Your cellular body has a powerful collective will-power to live and proactively defend both your life and their trillions-strong populated super colony.

- Your cellular body is highly ethical with each member willing to sacrifice itself to save the cellular colony that is your body; and in doing so saving your life and their own living super colony.

Despite how ancient the design of the human body is; the intelligence of your cells are medical genius beyond anything modern medicine can match or even still much even understand. Your cellular body is brilliant!

Each of us is unique. That is why in Chapters 9 & 10 on 35% Food Grade Hydrogen Peroxide internal super-oxygenation it is explained how you should let your body tell you how much your cellular body needs; rather than some set one- level-fits-all guideline. This is advice you will not find in most other books on hydrogen peroxide internal usage and super-oxygenation. It comes from the realization that your cellular body is vastly more intelligent than you, I or anyone else of what nutrients your cellular body uniquely needs; as you are a unique person.

Even a person's mental health, focus, emotions and psychological health are greatly and often decisively affected by the health of your cellular body.

The absolute and decisive truth is that your health and wellness - physical and psychological - is more dependent upon the health and power of your cellular body than any other factor. In fact, your very life depends upon them – the cells of your own body.

So it only makes sense that you eliminate chemicals, toxins and other substances that harm your cellular allies and friends. Give them all the vital oxygen and essential nutrients your cells need and use. Eliminate the chemicals and toxins in your life that weaken and harm your cells; as doing so equally is self-destruction.

If you do not, whose fault is it if your cellular body becomes too weak and fails you? They do so much for you, sacrifice themselves for you, and your life literally depends upon them.

Be good to your cells. Remember that the relationship between you and your trillions of cells is a 100% co-dependency for life itself. They are your best friend and your perfectly loyal ally.

This topic of organic metaphysics and communications between your conscious outer self and your inner cellular self it far too complex and would stray too much from direct focus to fully explore in this book.

I will not belabor the importance of not only providing your cellular body by providing sufficient oxygen and all vital nutrients, while eliminating toxins and other environmental damage, but also the importance of balance in your life for your overall true wellness. I am only reminding you what you already know.

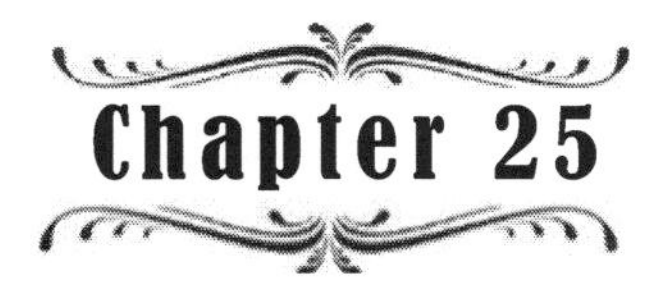

Chapter 25

Food For Thought

This may change how you perceive your goals for personal wellness.

> *What lies behind us and what lies before us are tiny matters... compared to what lies within us.*
>
> Ralph Waldo Emerson

We are all mortal and are destined to ultimately shipwreck. We all eventually will leave this life. The question then must be of the quality of life to the fullest. The quality, the effort, and the mentality of our life efforts should lead us to ask: What quality of ship is my life?"

We cannot return to the Garden of Eden nor can we obtain immortality in this lifetime. But now it is human-kind itself that evicts us further and further away from Eden.

So many people are looking for cures and answers; hope and solutions sought out in great and magical answers over the horizon – only to find countless claims by sellers of snake oil and with hope in invasive surgeries and debilitating pharmaceutical drugs. We want to believe the answer is "out there." Not inside us.

When the prescriptions, invasive procedures and surgeries fail, we then turn to allowing self-inflicted pain in radical physical therapies and intense self-denial of desires; believing somehow if we suffer enough we will be rewarded or believe that we are being punished for some sin or selfishness. We hope to endure this suffering, rather than continue to advance past it to overcome it.

If all that self-suffering also fails us, we slump our shoulders and resolve ourselves to the endless grind of life; we give up on ever solving the puzzle - attempting to replace defeating despair with acceptance of personal apathy about life. In the end, finally only waiting for relief by death, we hope that it will not be too painful. When a person lays down in acceptance, death will come even while still alive. Ultimately, we have diminished ourselves more than the disease has.

We should fully disagree to such defeat, but instead look to the origins-to the single cell of life itself - and the single cells of our own body. While I am my thoughts, I am dependent upon my body and my body is my cells. I demand so much from those cells; surely I should at least show them some respect for what they do.

I cannot succeed, cannot win, cannot declare all I do and then blame "them" or "that" if my body fails; nor claim I am an ethical and compassionate person - if I give no worth to those cellular creatures, the cells of my own body. If I show respect and reverence for any creatures it should be the cells of my body. No other creatures are more loyal or serve me better than the single cell organisms acting in harmony within the organs, bones and blood of my own body. Yet they are often only abused and neglected in return by us.

The most powerful microscopes still struggle to capture and understand the complexity of a single cell. Stronger microscopes continue to find the next layers of complexity. Human cells are not amoebas. They possess vastly complex internal structures, conduct amazing chemical processes of digestion, feeding, magnetic fields, memory, inter-relationship communication with each other, and collective effort.

No one has a clue how they decide, determine, adjust, communicate with each other, how the immune system remembers how to destroy previous viruses, reasons out problems or realize the environment around them. With each discovery more of the miracle of the human cell is revealed.

All living organisms are subject to tumors and have life spans. Even plants get tumors. But what determines how fast our life clock runs and in which direction? Which plants or animals will fall to tumors and which ones will not? Some biochemists now believed that human life could be increased to hundreds of years and cellular diseases virtually eliminated within a decade if this phenomenon is researched in depth.

In some ways this seems obvious. Our health and our life span are determined by cells of our body. Therefore, personal health focus should be at that level – cellular health.

Yes, these are mind boggling concepts. Yet I do not need to understand or accept a single word of it to understand that cellular health is decisively important to my health and well-being.

What our cellular body needs is a short and simple list. If all my body requires is oxygen, water, food, minerals, vitamins, a few amino acids and other fundamental organic nutrients, why would I refuse? I am too busy? It is too much of a bother? I cannot afford to feed them for pennies a day?

The reality of the cells of my body is that "They" are "I".

So I have decided to attempt to never deny the cells of my own body anything they need that I can attain or learn of. Not one element, not one mineral, not one atom or molecule will be held back from them. I will put on their menu plate what they wish - just as I do for myself. Just as my cells endlessly strive to figure out how to best to serve me by trial and error; so I now do the same for them.

How carelessly we abuse our bodies. We breathe poisons, eat toxins in our food, and swim in pools with toxic chemicals. We say "supersize it" to a meal of bleached flour without any value, grease, steroids and antibiotics in the meat, processed salt, sugar, artificial food dyes, starch and empty calories. A chemical diet drink or diet pill as our statement of health. Not 1% of the population looks at a menu or shops at the grocery store with the question, "What is truly good for me? What is not?"

We consider eating junk food as "treating ourselves", when that treat is worse than what we feed cattle and chickens or the cheapest dog food on the shelf. We will spend $5 for a burger, fries and a coke - at extreme prices - but will not pay the extra dime for an organically grown apple. We live and die on processed corn syrup carbonated water, chemical colors, starch, and fat as our daily diet. Maybe, just maybe, a person will take a ten cent vitamin pill once in a while believing this is sufficient.

When our bodies fail us - and they will - we hope a professional can give us the answer to the horrifying bad report of our fate in the doctor's office. We lament "Why me? What did I do to deserve this?" as though illness is a question of fairness or punishment - or just bad luck. Yet luck, fairness and punishment are not factors at all.

Yet it is not accurate to we claim it is nobody's fault.

Fault lies in agencies that certify unwholesome meat, milk, treated tap water and approve of the increasing levels of chemicals and toxins in our diet as "safe" and even "certified" and "inspected." Fault lies in health standards that allow putting toxins, radiation, and DNA destroying compounds into our air, water, and soil declared “safe” based minimal survival, no consideration of quality of life and life span that does not take into account these variables.

Fault lies in many places.

The importance of nutrition has been known to the human race for thousands of years and long before it was known that such a thing as vitamins, minerals and amino acids even existed. It has been known medically and scientifically for centuries that many diseases and illnesses are a direct result of the lack of specific vitamins or minerals.

It was known hundreds of years ago that sailors will sicken if only on a meat and bread diet, for which fruit was brought along. It was known that lack of iodine causes gout. Lack of fruit and vegetables causes scurry. Even animals know to seek minerals.

The list of causes is long. But this most basic fact of health that is fully solved for pennies a day has been ignored by a drug industry whose goal is to find the most expensive prescription drugs that the company can hold exclusive patent rights to, thus allowing astronomical profits. The profit motive system is that what is most profitable is what dictates policy, not whether it is beneficial to our health.

To listen carefully to the advertisements for many such artificial drugs is to realize that while promising it may offer one benefit it also warns of a dozen ways the drug can ruin your health or cost you your life. An expensive prescription drug is advertised as making a woman’s eye lashes grow longer – and then warns it can cause permanent blindness, facial distortion, kidney failure, stroke, heart attack and death. Are people that foolish and vulnerable to product marketing to gamble their body that way?

Fault lies in us, the people, for not expressing more gratitude and support for those doctors, scientists and researchers in the

medical field who do focus on health care as their priority - not personal profit - often making real economic and personal sacrifices to do so. Fault lies in us, the people, for not taking the time to search out such medical professionals.

Fault lies in the school cafeteria line, with menus planned upon a mix of what is the cheapest way to feed children food they will eat, rather than wholesome food. Fault lies in teaching that the measure of food is solely a measure of calories and listening to incessant advertising that junk food is treating and rewarding ourselves.

Fault lies in corporate farming on government policies that eliminates small family farms and upon the government encouraging same-crop usage of the identical land year after decade; and in tolerating - even certifying - the mass usage of steroid and antibiotics in meats of all kinds, and in allowing the selling of meats from diseased livestock.

Fault lies in our chemical industries and manufacturers within an economic political system that defined levels of extreme toxins and pathogens as "safe" levels in our food, products, air, water and environment. Fault lies in subsidized drug companies that define the best medicines are the most expensive drugs regardless of harms they cause.

Fault lies with us, the people, for not drawing distinction between the good and responsible chemical industries and the bad ones; good and bad politicians, and for paying little attention to such issues. Fault lies with politicians for not making distinction between regulations needed for our health and environment; compared to those that are bureaucratic harassment of honest companies.

Fault mostly lies in each of us for neglecting and abusing our own bodies. We know we should have eaten better and taken better care of ourselves. Fault lies in acceptance of "it's too late" in the face of serious medical illness. Yet with all this said, assigning fault is not a cure.

When ill, go to the doctor. Listen to your doctor's advice. But it also would be wise to look in the mirror and ask, "What should I do for myself?"

It is you, not the doctor, who will bear the consequences of the decisions that are yours to make. Thus, these are your decision. Decisions on how to avoid becoming ill. Decisions you make when you become ill also are your decisions.

A diagnosis of a terrible or fatal illness can lead to moments of deep feelings of loneliness and helplessness. The more crowded our world and lives become, the lonelier it seems people have become. Yet in that battle, you are not alone.

Tens of trillions of living and breathing creatures, your cells, are completely on your side with perfect loyalty and commonality of interests with you. They are fighting for you with all the power you allow them to have. They are completely depending upon you winning the battle for life, just as you are dependent upon them.

When it comes to fighting disease and physical failure, the truth is that they are more knowledgeable than anyone can comprehend - as that is their sole purpose of existence: To fight and even die if need in fighting to keep you alive and well. So for those reasons, be good to them – the cells of your own body.

Increasingly, I have come to realize that much of life, and of the world, is not out there but inside of myself.

The greatest and most decisive battles in my life are the ones I cannot see. The battles of my cells slaughtering virus, bacteria, fungus and defective cells by the billions - every day, every night - as our industrial world of toxic chemicals, worthless foods, declining oxygen levels in our air and radiation increasingly join forces to defeat my cellular armies and further degrade Eden.

The enemy hordes against my body are relentless. No matter

what stock I buy, what clothes I wear and what books I read, my whole life is dependent upon my cellular army winning every battle and every war.

Yet if we enter that world of those consumers blindly running from tent to tent of pitch men and marathon TV infomercials all hawking miracles in bottles of pills, who is being the fool? Who would even listen in that market place of foolishness but foolish people?

As our species races to ever more destroy the little left of our Eden, I yearn to return to the Garden. Maybe that too, is an inner cry of my cellular friends - they want to go home from where they first came.

Personally, I give credit for my existence - my soul and inner voice of self-realization - to my God. But for everything else of this life, I give credit to my cells. Without them, I am evicted from this life and reality.

No, I do not lotus position meditate in communion with my cells, though maybe it wouldn't hurt once in a while. I have been in discussions with others who claim human cells do not qualify as a living creatures because they do not think - as if anyone has a clue whether they do or not - as if this makes any difference to the issue.

This is what I know is true of my cells. If they lose, I lose.

This is the truism of each person's life. Every conscious effort of my life is reduced to nothingness if my cells lose a decisive battle with one a lethal tumor cell, lethal virus or degenerative disease.

As the cells of my own cellular body system sacrifice themselves without hesitation by the billions for me, maybe as an ethical person I should pause for a moment now and then and give them a thank you. As much as I admire the noble whale and worry of their future, should I not admire and worry more of those cellular creatures with in me – the trillions of cells of my own body of such devotion to me?

Increasingly, my suspicion is that they are wiser than I am. My cellular body does not need my ideology to exist, but I am entirely dependent upon their wisdom for my existence to continue. Without them - the cells of my own body - I cannot exist. Without the success of my cellular body, I will be evicted from this life. Therefore, they are important."

The above is anonymous copyrighted contribution cited in this book by copyright permission.

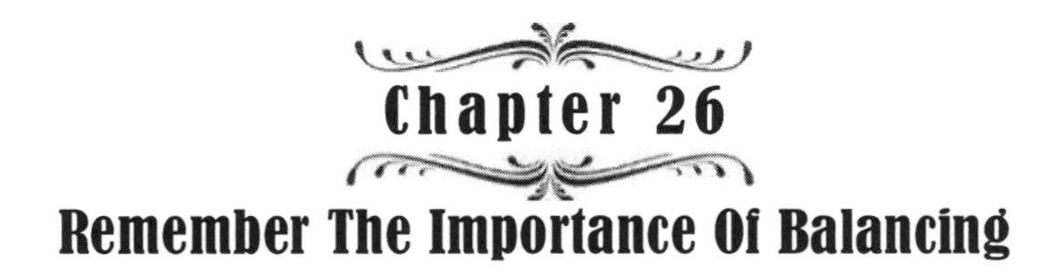

Chapter 26

Remember The Importance Of Balancing

Most people neglect personal healthcare and wellness. Even less consider the importance of cellular health and the importance of supplying your cellular body all the oxygen and vital nutrients they need in both to a total and balanced level.

Because you have this book and have reached this point in it, you are not such a person.

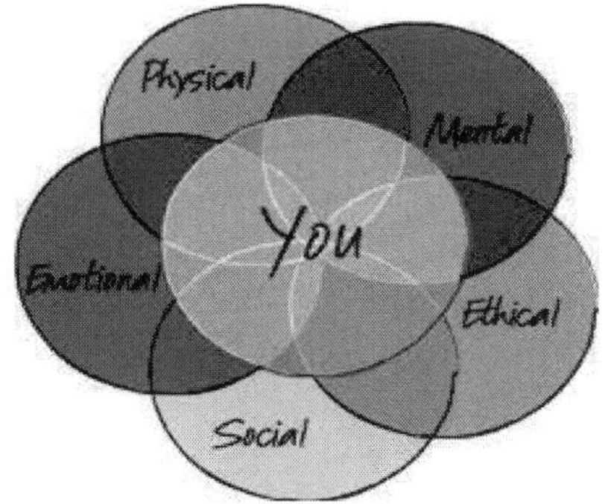

As you advance and benefit in your pursuit of true physical wellness in a harmony with your cellular-self and a fully complete and balanced manner, do not become so fixated on physical health that you forget the importance of the balance of your whole life.

If you wait until you are ready, you will be waiting for the rest of your life. The secret key to physical wellness is the pursuit of perfect cellular balance by providing of all the essential elements of life that your cellular body needs; while also protecting against invasive and destructive chemicals, pathogens, corrosives and cancer-causing agents internally and against your skin.

Health and Cheerfulness Naturally Beget Each Other

As you pursue and achieve cellular health and physical wellness, do not neglect the essential balance of your whole life; nor make physical health become of such great importance you forget the greater overall priorities in life.

The key to WELLNESS is to accept personal responsibility for your health & wellbeing.

Do not delay the other needs for your Wellness of Life. The secret key to true total wellness in life is the greater balancing of your whole life to obtain true total personal wellness.

Learn & Sharing Increasing Knowledge

If you would like to receive updates and additional information and knowledge as it becomes known and discovered - and to share in the knowledge, experiences and discoveries of others - from experts to other good folks such as yourself - send an email to the author just writing "put me on your updating list" to:

PowerOfHydrogenPeroxide@gmail.com

The author invites you to share your knowledge, experiences and discoveries with her and with others through her.

Author's Closing Comment

Thank you so very much for spending time with this book. For any information, advice or steps to follow that you determine is worthwhile, convey it to others so they can benefit too.

If you have a spare minute, drop me an email with your comments and your own views on any of these topics:

PowerOfHydrogenPeroxide@gmail.com

It has been the great sharing of information, whether one-to-one or worldwide, that is now opening so many eyes and minds to the true miracle path to natural whole wellness. I hope to hear from you.

I wish you and your loved ones the very best of that life has to offer.

Mary

Bibliography & Resources List

Ackerman N B, Brinkley F B: Comparison of Effect son Tissue Oxygenation of Hyperbaric Oxygen and Intravascular Hydrogen Peroxide.Sur.1968; 63: 285-290

Archibald F S and Duong M N: Superoxide Dismutase and Oxygen

Toxicity Defenses in the Genus Neisseria. 1986;

Arteriosclerosis, Saito N/Nippon Rinsho (JAPAN) Jan 1996, 54 (1) p59-66

Balla, G.A.; Finney, J.W.; Aronoff, B.L. et all: Use of Intra-arterial Hydrogen Peroxide to Promote Wound Healing. Amr. J. Surergyl 1964; 108:621-629

Belotskii S M, Filiudova OB, Pashutin S B, et al: Chemiluminescence of Human Neutrophils as Affected by Opportunistic Microbes. Zh. Mikrobiol. Epidemiol. Immunobiol.m1986; Mar (3): 89-92

Brandi G, Sestili P, Pedrini M A, et al: The Effect of Temperature or Anoxia on Escherichia Coli KillingInduced by Hydrogen Peroxide. Mutat Res. 1987;190(4): 23740

Brinkmann V, Kaufmann S H, Simon M M, et al: Role of Macrophages in Malaria: 02 Metabolite Production and Phagocytosis by Splenic Macrophages During Lethal Plasmodium berghei and Self-limiting Plasmodium yoelii Infection in Mice.1984; 44(3): 7434. Biochem.Biophys. Res. Commun. 1985: 127(1): 270-6.100.Pruitt Km, Tenovuo J, Mansson-Rahemtulla B, et al: Is Thiocyanate Peroxidation at Equilibrium In-Vivo? Biochem. Biophys. Acta 1986; 870(3):

Burke T M and Wolin M S: Hydrogen Peroxide Elicits Pulmonary Artery Relaxation and Guanylate Cyclase Activation. Am. J. Physiol. 1987; 252(4 Pt 2): H721-32

Calcium, phosphorus and magnesium intakes correlate with bone mineral content in postmenopausal women, GYNECOL. ENDOCRINOL. (United Kingdom), 1994, 8/1 (55-58)

Chlorine Dangers, PhD biologist/chemist Dr. Herbert Schwartz 1997

Cranne D, Haussinger D, Sies H: Rise of CoenzymeA-Glutathione Mixed Disulfide during Hydro-peroxide Metabolism in Perfused Rat Liver. Euo. J.Biochem. 1982; 127: 575-578.

Comparative findings on serum IMg2+ of normal and diseased human subjects with the NOVA and KONE ISE's for Mg2+, SCAND. J. CLIN. LAB. INVEST. SUPPL. (United Kingdom), 1994, 54/217

Derivatives of Bacterial Components in Bacterial Action against Eschericia coli. 1979;23: 522- 531

"The Dead Sea" National Psoriasis Foundation. Retrieved on 2008-04-10. The susceptibility of the centrocecal scotoma to electrolytes, especially in multiple sclerosis, IDEGGYOG.SZLE (HUNGARY), 1973, 26/7 (307-312) Thomas EL: Myeloperoxidase, Hydrogen Peroxide, Chloride Antimicrobial System: Nitrogen-Chlorine

Del Maestro RF, Thaw H H, Bjork J, et al: Free Radicals as Mediators of Tissue Injury. Acta Physiol.Scand. 1980; 492 (supple): 43-57

Didenko W: Possible Role of Lipid Peroxidation inthe Pathogenesis of Arrhythmias in Myocardial Infarct. Biull. Eksp. Biol. Med. 1985; 99(6): 647-9

Diez-Marques M L, Lucio-Cazana F J and Rodriguez Puyol M: InVitro Response of Erythrocytes to Alphatocopherol Exposure. Int. J. Vita., Nutr., Res1986; 56(3): 311-315.

Disorders of magnesium metabolism, Endocrinology and Metabolism Clinics of North America (USA), 1995, 24/3

Dockrell H M and Play fair J H: Killing of Blood-Stage Murine Malaria Parasites by Hydrogen Peroxide.

Doroshow J H: Role of Hydrogen Peroxide and Hydroxyl Radical Formation in the Killing of Ehrlich Tumor Cells by Anticancer Quinones. Proc. Natl.Acad. Sci. USA 986; 83(12): 4514-8

Douglas, William Campbell, M.D. Hydrogen Peroxide Medical Miracle, Clayton GA 30525

Ehrhardt, Proksch; Nissen, HP; Bremgartner, M; Urquhart, C. "Bathing in a magnesium-rich Dead Sea salt solution: follow-on review". International Journal of Dermatology 46 (2): 177–179. doi:10.1111/j.1365-4632.2005.02079.x. PMID 15689218.

Eilin P J, Strulowitz J A, Wolin M S, et al: Absence of a Role for Superoxide Anion, Hydrogen Peroxide and Hydroxyl Radical in Endothelium mediated Relaxation of Rabbit Aorta. Electromyographical ischemic test and intracellular and extracellular magnesium concentration in migraine and tension-type headache patients, HEADACHE (UNITED STATES) Jun 1996, 36 (6) p357-61

Energy and nutrient intake in patients with CF, Monatsschrift fur
Kinderheilkunde (Germany), 1996, 144/4 (396-402)

Experimental and clinical studies on dysregulation of magnesium metabolism and the aetiopathogenesis of multiple sclerosis, Magnes Res (ENGLAND) Dec 1992, 5 (4) p295-302

Farr, C H, Physiological and Biochemical Responses to Intravenous Hydrogen Peroxide in Man, J ACMA 1987

Farr, C H, The Therapeutic Use of Intravenous Hydrogen Peroxide, 1987

Ferrante A, Hill N L Abell TJ, et al: Role of Myelo-peroxidase in the Killing of Naegleria fowleri byLymphokine-altered Human Neutrophils. 1987; 55(5):1047-50.86.

Finney J W, Balla G A, Race GJ, et al: Peripheral Blood Changes in Humans and Experimental Animals Following the Infusion of Hydrogen Peroxide into the Carotid Artery. Angio 1965

Finney JW, Jay B E, Race G J, et al: Removal of Cholesterol and Other Lipids from Experimental Animal and Human Atheromatous Arteries by Dilute Hydrogen Peroxide. Angiology 1966; 17: 223-228.

Finney J W, Urschel HC, Balla GA, et al: Protection of the Ischemic Heart with DMSO Alone or DMSO with Hydrogen Peroxide. Ann. NY Acad. Sci. 1967;151: 231-241.

Florence T M127: The Degradation of Cytochrome C by Hydrogen Peroxide. J. Inorg. Biochem. 1985; 23(a):132-41.

Fontanarosa, Phil (2002). Alternative Medicine: An Objective Assessment. New York: American Medical Association. p. 112. ISBN 1-57947-002-5.

Fuson R L, Kylstra J A, Hochstein P, et al: Intravenous Hydrogen Peroxide Infusion as a Means of Extra-pulmonary Oxygenation. Clin. Res.1967

Garner M H, Garner W H, Spector A: Kinetic Cooperativity Change after H2O2 Modification of (Na,K)-ATPase, J. Biolog. Chem. 1984; 259: 7712-7718.

Germon P A, Faust DS, Brady, LW: Comparison of Arterial and Tissue Oxygen Measurements in Hu-mans Receiving Regional Hydrogen Peroxide Infu-sions and Oxygen Inhalation. Radiology 1968; 91:669-672

Germon P A, Faust DS, Rosenthal A, et al: Regional Arterial and Tissue Oxygen Tensions in Man Dur-ing Regional Infusion with Hydrogen Peroxide Solutions. Radiology 1967; 88:589-591

Ghadirian E, Somerfield SD, Kongshavn PA: Sus-ceptibility of Entamoeba Histolytica to Oxidants.1985; 51 (1): 263-7

Gorren AC, Dekker H and Weaver R: Kinetic Investigations of the Reactions of Cytochrome C Oxidase with Hydrogen Peroxide. Biochem. Biophys. Acta.1986; 852(1): 81-95.

Gutteridge J M and Wilkins S: Copper Salt-depen-dent Hydroxyl Radical Formation. Damage to pro-teins Acting as Antioxidants. Biochim. Beefiest. Acta 1983; 759(1-2): 38-41

Harari, Marco; Shani, Jashovam. "Demographic evaluation of successful antipsoriatic climatotherapy at the Dead Sea (Israel) DMZ Clinic". International Journal of Dermatology 36 (4): 304–305. doi:10.1046/j.1365-4362.1997.00204.x.

Harrison J F and Schultz J: Studies on the Chlorinating Activity of Myeloperoxidase Biol. Chem. 1976; 251:13711374.

Helm A U and Gunn J: The Effect of Insulino mimetic Agents on Protein Degradation in H-35 Hepatoma Cells. Mol. Cell. Biochem.1986; 71(2): 159-166.

Hofmann C, Crettas M, Burns P, et al: Cellular Responses Elicited by Insulin Mimickers in Cells Lacking Detectable Plasma Membrane Insulin Receptors. J. Cell. Biochem. 1985; 27(4): 401-14.

Howells RE: The Modes of Action of Some Anti-protozoal Drugs. Parasitology 1985

Hypocalcemia associated with estrogen therapy for metastatic adenocarcinoma of the prostate, J. UROL. (USA), 1988, 140/5 PART I (1025-1027)

Looney R J and Steigbigel R T: Role of the Vi Antigen of Salmonella typhi in Resistance to Host Defense In Vitro. J. Lab. Clin. Med. 1986; 108(5): 506-16.

Jay B E, Finney JW, Balla G A, et al. The Supersaturation of Bio logic Fluids with Oxygen by the Decom-position of Hydrogen Peroxide. Texas Rpts. Bio l and Med 1964; 106-109

Jepras R I and Fitzgeorge R B: The Effect of Oxygen-dependent Ant imicrobial Systems on Strains of Legionella Pneumophila of Different Virulence. J.Hyg. (Lond) 1986; 97(1):61-9.

Johnson R J R, Froese G, Khodadad M, et al: Hydrogen Peroxide and radiotherapy. Bubble Formation in Blood. Br. J. Radio l. 1968; 41: 749-754

Kidney stone clinic: Ten years of experience, Nederlands Tijschrift voor de Klinische Chemie (Netherlands), 1996, 21/1 (8-10)

Kiebanoff S J: Oxygen Metabolism and the Toxic Properties of Phagocytes. Ann. Intern. Med. 1980; 93:480-489.55.Slivka A, LoBuglio AF, Weiss SJ: A Potential Role for Hypochlorous Acid in Granulocyte-Mediated Tumor Cell Toxicity. Blood 1980 347-350

Klebanoff S J and Shepard C C: Toxic Effect of thePeroxidase-hydrogen peroxide-halide Antimicrobial System on Mycobacterium leprae. 1984; 44(2): 534

Kontos H A: Oxygen Radicals in Cerebral Vascular Injury. Circ. Res.m1985; 57(4): 508-16.

Magnesium deficiency and sudden death, S. AFR. MED. J. (SOUTH AFRICA), 1983, 64/18 (697-698)

Magnesium deficiency produces spasms of coronary arteries: Relationship to etiology of sudden death ischemic heart disease, SCIENCE (USA), 1980, 208/4440 (198-200)

Magnesium and potassium in diabetes and carbohydrate metabolism. Review of the present status and recent results, Magnesium 1984. 3(4-6). P 315-23

Magnesium in the physiopathology and treatment of renal calcium stones, PRESSE MED. (FRANCE), 1987, 16/1 (25-27)

Magnesium supplementation and osteoporosis, Nutrition Reviews (USA), 1995, 53/3 (71-74)

MacNaughton JI: Regional Oxygenation and Radio-therapy: A Study of the Degradation of Infused Hydrogen Peroxide. I. Infusate Mixing. Int. J. Radiat.Biol. 1971

McCabe, Ed; Oxygen Therapies, Morrisville, NY 12408, 1990

Meyer CT, Brand M, DeLuca VA,e t al; Hydrogen Peroxide Colitis: A Report of Three Patients. J. Clin Gastroenterol 1981; 3:31-35.

Migraine--diagnosis, differential diagnosis and therapy, Ther Umsch (SWITZERLAND) Feb 1997, 54 (2) p64-70

Minotti G and Aust SD: The Requirement for Iron (III) in the Initiation of Lipid Peroxidation byIron(II) and Hydrogen Peroxide. J. Biol. Chem. 1987:262(3):1098-104.

Moran A P and Upton M E: Effect of Medium Supplements, Illumination and Superoxide Dismutaseon the Production of Coccoid Forms of Campy-lobacter jejuni ATCC29428. J. Appl. Bacteriol. 987;62(1): 43-51.

Nathan, C F; Cohn Z A; Antitumor Effects of Hydrogen Peroxide in Vivo, J. Exp. Med. 1981; 154: 1529-1553

Magnesium concentration in plasma and erythrocytes in MS, Acta Neurologica Scandinavica (Denmark), 1995, 92/1 (109-111)

Magnesium and the premenstrual syndrome, ANN. CLIN. BIOCHEM. (UK), 1986, 23/6 (667-670)

Magnesium concentration in brains from multiple sclerosis patients, ACTA NEUROL. SCAND. (Denmark), 1990, 81/3 (197-200)

Magnesium deficiency produces insulin resistance and increased thromboxane synthesis, HYPERTENSION (USA), 1993, 21/6 II (1024-1029)

Magnesium and glucose homeostasis, DIABETOLOGIA (Germany, Federal Republic of), 1990, 33/9 (511-514)

Magnesium content of erythrocytes in patients with vasospastic angina, CARDIOVASC. DRUGS THER. (USA), 1991, 5/4 (677-680)

Magnesium deficiency: Possible role in osteoporosis associated with gluten-sensitive enteropathy, Osteoporosis International (United Kingdom), 1996, 6/6 (453-461)

Magnesium and carbohydrate metabolism, THERAPIE (France), 1994, 49/1 (1-7)

Magnesium hormonal regulation and metabolic interrelations, PRESSE MED. (France), 1988, 17/12 (584-587)

Marshall PJ and Lands W E: In Vitro Formation of Activators for Prostaglandin Synthesis by Neutrophils and Macrophages from Humans and Guinea Pigs. J. Lab. Clin. Med.1986; 108 (6) :525-534

Miller S A, Bia F J, Coleman D L, et al: Pulmonary Macrophage Function During Experimental Cytomegalovirus Interstitial Pneumonia. 1985; 47(1): 211-6

Miyasaki K T, Wilson M E, Genco R J: Killing of Actinobacillus actinomycetemcomitans by the Human Neutrophil Myeloperoxidase-hydrogen peroxide-chloride System. 1986; 53(1): 161-5

Murray HW, Scavuzzo D., Jacobs JL, et al: In Vitroand In Vivo Activation of Human MononuclearPhagocytes by Interferon-gamma. Studies withNormal and AIDS Monocytes. J. 2987;138(8): 2457-62

Murray HW: Cellular Resistance to Protozoal Infection. Annu. Rev. Med.1986; 37: 61-9

Nelson D H and Murray D K: Dexamethasone Inhibition of Hydrogen Peroxide stimulated Glucose Transport Endocrinology 1987; 120(1): 156-159.

Oral magnesium successfully relieves premenstrual mood changes, OBSTET. GYNECOL. (USA), 1991, 78/2 (177-181)

Norkus E P, Kuenzig W, Conney A H: Studies on the Mutagenic Activity of Ascorbic Acid in Vitro and in Vivo. Mutat. Res. 1983; 117(1): 183-9

Oliver T H, Cantab B C, and Murphy DV: Influenzal Pneumonia: The Intravenous Injection of Hydrogen Peroxide.Lancet 1920; 1: 432-433.

Oya Y, Yamamoto K, Tonomura A: The Biological Activity of Hydrogen Peroxide. 1. Induction of Chromosome-type Aberrations Susceptible to Inhi-bition by Scavangers of Hydroxyl Radicals in Human Embryonic Fibroblasts. 1986;172(3): 245-53.103.

Proksch, Ehrhardt MD, PhD et al. "Bathing in a magnesium-rich Dead Sea salt solution improves skin barrier function, enhances skin hydration, and reduces inflammation in atopic dry skin", International Journal of Dermatology, February 2005. Retrieved on 2008-04-13.

Paget TA, Fry M, Lloyd D: Effects of Inhibitors onthe Oxygen Kinetics of Nippostrongylus brasiliensis. Mol. Biochem. Parasitol. 1987; 22(2-3): 125-33

Plasma copper, zinc and magnesium levels in patients with premenstrual tension syndrome, ACTA OBSTET. GYNECOL. SCAND. (Denmark), 1994, 73/6 (452-455)

Podoplekina LE, Shutova NA, Fyodorov YuV: Influ-ence of Several Chemical Reagents on LymphocyticChoriomeningitis and Tacaribe Viruses. Virologie 1986; 37(1): 43-8

Prophylaxis of migraine with oral magnesium: results from a prospective, multi-center, placebo-controlled and double-blind randomized study, Cephalalgia (NORWAY) Jun 1996, 16 (4) p257-63

Ramasarma T: Generation of H2O2 in Biomembranes. Biochemica et Biophysica ACTA 1982; 694: 69-93.

Renal stone formation in patients with inflammatory bowel disease, SCANNING MICROSC. (USA), 1993, 7/1 (371-380)

Rilling, Siegfried, MD; Viebahn, Renate, Ph.D.; The Use of Ozone in Medicine. Heidelberg, Germany 1987

Root R K, Metcalf J A, Oshino N, et al: H2O2 Release from Human Granulocytes during Phagocytosis. J.Clin. Invest.1975; 55:945-955. Root R K and Metcalf J A: H2O2 MIRACLE man Granulocytes during Phagocytosis. 1977 ;60: 1266-1279.

Rothermel C D, Rubin BY, Jaffe EA, et al: Oxygen-in-dependent Inhibit ion of Intracellular Chlamydiapsittaci Growth by Human Monocytes and Interferon-gamma-activated Macrophages. J.1986; 137(2): 689

Rotstein O D, Nasmith P E, Grinstein S: The Bacteroides Byproduct Succinic Acid Inhibits Neutro-phil Respiratory Burst by Reducing Intracellular pH. 1987; 55(4): 864-70.

Rubanyi GM and Vanhoutte PM: Oxygen-derivedFree Radicals, Endothelium and Responsiveness of Vascular Smooth Muscle. Am. J. Physiol. 1986; 250(5pt 2): H815-821.

Schaffner A, Davis C E, Schaffner T, et al: In Vitro Susceptibility of Fungi to Killing by Neutrophil Granulocytes Discriminates Between Primary Pathogenicity and Opportunism. J. 1986;

Scott J A, Fischman A J, Khaw BA, et al: Free Radica lMediated Membrane Depolarizat ion in Renal andCardiac Cells. Biochim. Biophys. Acta 1987; 899(1):76-82

Shah J, Pedemonte M S, Wilcock M M: Hydrogen Peroxide May Cause Venous Oxygen Embolism Anesthesiology 1984; 61:631-632.

Shenep JL, Stokes D C, Hughes W T: Lack of Antibacterial Activity After Intravenous Hydrogen Peroxide Infusion in Experimental Escherichia coli Sepses. 1985; 48:607-610.7.

Shimada O and Yashuda H: Lipid Peroxidation and its Inhibition by Tinoridine. Biochem. Biophys. ACTA 1979; 572:531

Shingu M, Yoshioka K, Nobunaga M, et al: HumanVascular Smoothare Susceptible to Hydrogen Peroxide. Inflammation 1985; 9(3): 309-320.98.

Sleigh J, Linter S P K: Hazards of Hydrogen Peroxide.1985; 291:1706.

Statement of Theory, Guardian of Eden, 13-23, 2008

Steiner B M, Wong G H, Sutrave P, et al: Oxygen Toxicity in Treponema Pallidum: Deoxyribonucleic Acid Single stranded Breakage Induced by Low Doses of Hydrogen Peroxide. Can. J. Microbiol.1984;30 (12): 1467-76

Swaroop A and Ramasarma T: Heat Exposure and Hypothyroid Conditions Decrease Hydrogen Peroxide Production Generation in Liver Mitochrondia. J. Biochem. 1985; 226(2): 403-8.

Super Nutrition for Healthy Hearts, Dr. Richard Passwater

Tappel A L: Lipid Peroxidation Damage to Cell Component. Fed Proc. 1973; 32:1870

Tenovuo J, Makinen K, Sievers G: Antibacterial Ef-fect of Lactoperoxidase and MyeloperoxidaseAgainst Bacillus cereus. Antimicrob. Agents Che-mother. 1985; 27(1): 96-101.

Toxicity of chlorine, Dr. Stephen Askin 2003

Tsan M F, Danis E H, Del Vecchio P J, et al: Enhancement of Intracellular Gluthathione Protects Endothelial Cells Against Oxidant Damage. Biochem. Beefiest. Res. Commun. 1985: 127(1): 270-6.

Variant angina due to deficiency of intracellular magnesium, CLIN. CARDIOL. (USA), 1990, 13/9 (663-665)

Urinary factors of kidney stone formation in patients with Crohn's disease, KLIN. WOCHENSCHR. (Germany, Federal Republic of), 1988, 66/3 (87-91)

Urschel H E Jr: Cardiovascular Effects of Hydrogen Peroxide: Current Status. Dis. of Chest 1967;51:180192.

Urschel H C, Finney JW, Morale AR, et al: Cardiac Resuscitation with Hydrogen Peroxide. Circ. 1965;31 (suppl II); II-210.

Usage of 35% Food Grade Hydrogen Peroxide, Guardian of Eden, 1-7, 2012

Verhoeven A J, Mommersteeg M E, Akkerman J W: Balanced Contribution of Glycolyte and Adenylate Pool in Supply of Metabolic Energy.

Ward J F, Blakey W F, Joner El: Mammalian Cells arenot Killed by DNA Single-strand Breaks Caused by Hydroxyl Radicals from Hydrogen Peroxide Endothelial Cells Against Oxidant Damage

Wei E P, Christman C W, Kontos H A, et al: Effects of Oxygen Radicals on Cerebral Arterioles. Am J Physiol 1985; 248(2 pt 2): H157-62 Platelets. J. Biol.Chem. 1985; 260(5): 2621-4.

Weiss SJ, Young J, LoBuglio A, et al: Role of Hydrogen Peroxide in Neutrophil-Mediated Destruction of Cultured Endothelial Cells. 1981; 68:714-721.

Wildberger E, Kohler H, Jenzer H, et al: Inactivation of Peroxidase and Glucose Oxidase by H2O2 and Iodide during In Vitro Thyroglobulin Iodination. Mol Cell Endocrinol 1986; 46(2): 149-154.

Wrigglesworth JM: Formation and Reduction of a 'Peroxy' Intermediate of Cytochrome C Oxidase by Hydrogen Peroxide. Biochem. J. 1984; 217; 715-719

Zaizen Y, Nakagawara A, Ikeda K: Patterns of Destruction of Mouse Neuroblastoma Cells by Extracellular Hydrogen Peroxide Formed by 6-hydroxydopamine and Ascorbate. J. Cancer Res.Clin. Oncol. 1986; 111(2):93-7

Zgliczynski J M, Selvaraj RJ, Paul B B, et at Chlorination by the Myeloperoxidase-H202-Cl antimicrobial system at Acid and Neutral pH. Soc. Exp. Bioi Med. 1977; 154: 418422.

Zinc, copper and magnesium concentration in serum and CSF of patients with neurological disorders, ACTA NEUROL. SCAND. (Denmark), 1989, 79/5 (373-378)

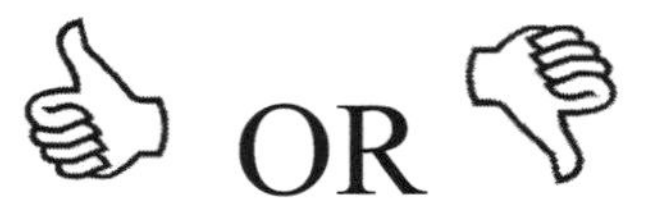

What is your vote on this book?

The author invites your opinions, suggestions
& personal health and wellness experiences

PowerOfHydrogenPeroxide@gmail.com
Attn: Mary

To check for new information or updates visit
PowerOfHydrogenPeroxide.com/updates.htm

If you would like to order a copy for a friend visit
PowerOfHydrogenPeroxide.com/book.htm